Red Cross
and
Iron Cross

by
Axel Munthe

© 2008 Benediction Classics, Oxford. .

FOREWORD

FOREWORD

THE day of reckoning will come. The day when the civilized world sets to work to pick out the criminals from the barbarians, the criminals responsible for the atrocities and infamies committed by the savage foe. The documents for the accusation furnished by the accused themselves—a most valuable contribution to the sombre study of German criminology—establish beyond doubt that it is on the leaders and not on the men that the heaviest responsibility will fall. The hanging evidence against several of the commanding German Generals in Belgium is overwhelming—their proclamations to their victims and their orders to their troops contain damning proofs that they are morally and legally responsible for the slaughter of hundreds of helpless civilians, men, women and children. Accusations of instigation to murder, even of the wounded, are brought against officers of all ranks by their men in their note-books—now in the hands of the Belgian, French and English authorities. As to the men themselves, the writers of these precious human documents, most of them have already gone to their doom, and all we know of them are the horrors they have witnessed and the atrocities they have committed. Many are still alive and prisoners of war. Others have died in our ambulances side by side with their former foes, now their comrades in suffering and as often as not almost their friends. I have had some dealings with several of these men. I have read their note-books, I have heard from their own lips their gruesome tales of recorded and unrecorded horror. Those dying men told no lies. Man speaks the truth when he is aware that Death is listening to what he says.

Suffering has no nationality and Death wears no uniform. There are neither friends nor foes on " no-man's-land," on all men's land, on the borderland between life and death, dreaded by all. Men die as best they can. Most men fear death, all men fear dying. All men are more or less alike when they are about to die. What they did with their life whilst it belonged to them may concern the priest if he is at hand, but Death does not care, he welcomes them all in his own rough way, good men and bad men are all the same to him. So they are to the doctor. Now and then I tried to say to myself that I disliked these dying Boches, but I cannot honestly say I did; in fact, I rather liked them. These were all so forlorn, so patient, so humble, so grateful for the little one was able to do for them. They were all delighted to come across a man who knew their language—those who could smile grinned all over with joyous surprise, those who could not, greeted the familiar sound with a friendly look or a tear in their tired eyes. Those who could speak, or nearly all of them, spoke with humiliation and shame of what they had witnessed and what they had done. They certainly did not spare themselves; on the contrary, they seemed to like to talk of their evil deeds as if it gave them some relief—in fact, they did not want to talk of anything else. I saw several of these men die. They died as brave men die.

No one accustomed to the cheerful, affectionate way the French and English soldiers are wont to speak of their leaders, could avoid being struck by the way these German soldiers talked of their officers. They all spoke of them with fear and bitterness and often with hatred. Even as they lay there safe in one of our ambulances they seemed to be afraid of lying next to their own officers. Luckily this did not happen often and never for long, for the German officers always protested furiously against being placed with their own men. Besides, it mattered little where they were placed, they were invariably dissatisfied anyhow. Those I saw were sullen, arrogant and often insolent; displeased with everything and everybody and most difficult to deal with. They always spoke of their rank and their Iron Cross—unavoidable it seemed to me, as I never came across an officer without it— as if entitling them to privileges shared by no one else. They were well pleased with themselves and their doings, frightfulness and all, and never did I hear from any of them a word which sounded like disapproval of the atrocities they had witnessed. Personally I only know of one German officer who disapproves this frightfulness, and his mother was a Russian. On the contrary, I heard a captain say that the Belgians had been treated much too leniently, and that all the civil population ought to have been driven out of their country and those who resisted shot on the spot. This officer was a Prussian. The marked difference between Prussians and South Germans, well known to those who have visited Germany in times of peace, has been amply illustrated by the conduct of the different units in this war.

" The Prussian is cruel by birth, civilization will make him ferocious," said Goethe, who knew his country well. It is true that the French soldier always singles out the Bavarians as particularly brutal and violent and especially fond of looting; but I wonder if this evil reputation of theirs is not to a certain extent founded upon vague reminiscences from the war of '70. It must be admitted though that their record at Nomély, Blamont and several other places is a terrible one. But I do not forget that the unnamed hero of this little book was a Bavarian soldier.

It matters little that I could not identify the band of barbarians who had established themselves in the château mentioned in this book—similar scenes have occurred everywhere ever since the war began, and hundreds of châteaux in Belgium and France, have had a much worse fate. I admit though that when I wrote down the description of the devastated nursery I believed that this particularly revolting deed was unique of its kind. Not at all; I was mistaken. I have read since then from the pen of a distinguished English surgeon in Belgium a description of a similar act of incredible barbarism. But I am very sorry I do not know more of the German officer who after a prolonged contemplation in front of the Venetian mirror smashed it with a knock of his sword-hilt—the old caretaker just entered the drawing-room in time to witness this performance.

I am glad at least to be able to hail his comrade-in-arms, the Adalbert of this book, by his well-fitting Christian name; his family name was too long to remember, I have had to shorten it here for convenience sake. I know well he is a rather unusual type of German officer, but since I had the good luck to have half an hour's conversation with this phenomenon I do not see why I should not let the reader share the pleasure of his acquaintance. Moreover, I was told by Dr. Martin, who knew the Germans far better than I do, that after all Adalbert was not such an uncommon type of German officer as I seemed to think—I was delighted to hear it, so much the better for us. He wanted to know if I was a nobleman: *sind sie Adel?* He seemed to have his doubts about it. It would amply satisfy all my literary ambitions were I able to present him with this photograph of himself, slightly retouched by a lenient hand, but very like him. I wish I knew where he was, he ought not to be difficult to trace. Maybe " Potsdam " would find him . . .

But the others, the dear old village doctor, the white-haired Curé, Sœur Marthe and

Sœur Philippine, and Josephine with her kind brown eyes, where shall I find them? Their village is a heap of blackened ruins, four naked walls are all that remains of their church, and God knows where they are! God knows where they are. They are all over France, in every hamlet, every village and every town, soothing the sufferings of the wounded and sharing their bread with the homeless. Dr. Martin is dead. He was first reported missing and it was thought he had fallen into the hands of the Boches. He was soon afterwards found dead, with Josephine's medal round his neck. Better so for him. I am sure he would have preferred the second alternative had he had the choice.

But I am equally sure that Adalbert is not dead. I am sure he is still as fit and alert as when I saw him, safe under the protection of the law of irony—maybe I would have spared him had I doubted his invulnerability. Even so, as I read through this manuscript, my literary instinct, rudimentary though it may be, tells me that this Adalbert does not fit in very well in the "composition," if a layman may use such an expression. I am sure it would have been wiser to keep him to myself for fear that his harsh giggle might jar on the reader of this tale of suffering and woe. But life is made up of such contrasts and so is death. No, I know well he does not fit in the composition. Anyhow I shall leave him in the place where I found him, like the bell-capped buffoon strutting about amongst the swordsmen and arquebusiers on an old Flemish tapestry, or like the grinning monkey crouching in the corner of a primitive old painting of martyrs and saints. Yes, martyrs and saints they are indeed, the other figures I have tried to paint with loving hands on the remaining pages of this little book! Martyrs giving their lives for a sacred cause and saints bending over bleeding wounds and gently closing the eyes of the dead with prayers on their lips. The background of the picture is the fair land of France with its devastated plains and its ruined homes, and far away against the reddening sky Rheims Cathedral in flames! Brave and chivalrous France, so calm in her hour of danger, so dignified in her sorrow, so strong in the consciousness of her unconquerable soul.

* *

I just caught a glimpse of a handful of Tommies as they flung themselves into the midst of the fray to fight the Hun by the side of their dauntless ally. I heard them singing and laughing in their water-logged trenches in Flanders, and I saw them, agile as leopards, leap from their parapets and, led by a boy officer swinging his cane, spring forward to meet death half-way as joyously as though to welcome a friend.

I know that Tommy will play the game, it is the game he has played so often and played so well, it is the old game between Right and Wrong!

I know what stuff he is made of, that mighty fighter; I know that his heart is sound and that his arm is strong. Strike hard, Tommy, strike your hardest! It is the salvation of the world you are fighting for! I have known all along that you were coming. I have known it ever since I was a boy and began to read the History of England! I have known it all along, but God bless you all the same, Tommy, for coming! And God be thanked that you came!

I

RED CROSS AND IRON CROSS

I

THE stranger walked slowly down the narrow main street stretching from one end of the village to the other. Some of the houses were all in ruins, and in others the roof or a portion of the wall had fallen in. The road was covered with debris of bricks and plaster and strewn with broken glass. In the Square some children crawled out from under a broken-down transport wagon to gaze at the stranger as he passed, and further down the street two boys sat riding astride a gun-carriage with smashed wheels.

A glance at the inn took away his last hope of breakfast; a huge hole in the wall just over the porch showed only too clearly that the shell had done its work well, and that the whole fabric was on the point of tumbling to pieces at any moment. Here and there the anxious face of a woman looked out from a half-closed doorway, but otherwise all seemed deserted.

At the other end of the street stood the church on rising ground, and further on, as far as the eye could see, the usual poplar-lined French chaussée stretched away in one straight line towards the distant Eastern hills. The church looked undamaged, and so did the adjoining Presbytery in its little grove of elm-trees.

Outside the portal of the church stood the old curé, and at his side another old man who proved to be the mayor and the village doctor in one person, eyeing with uncomfortable curiosity the approaching stranger. The sight of the red ribbon on his dilapidated tunic removed their uneasiness at once, and when the stranger told them that he was a doctor and belonged to the British Red Cross they received him with open arms.

"It is God Himself who has sent you here, Dr. Martin," said the Curé in his kind voice.

The doctor did not look quite so sure of that, but was evidently pleased to be spared any explanation as to what had landed him there, with all his kit lost and nothing but a morphia syringe in his pocket and a packet of cigarettes and a little tea in his haversack.

"We are badly in need of help, *mon cher confrère*," said the old village doctor as they went in.

A heart-rending subdued moan filled the church with awe. On the straw-covered floor lay, side by side, over a hundred grievously wounded soldiers. They were all dying men, with blood-stained, mud-covered, greatcoats hiding ghastly wounds and torn limbs. Here and there the very straw was red, and streamlets of blood trickled slowly down the slippery marble floor. Here and there well-meaning but inexperienced hands had tried to stem the hæmorrhage or to cover a gaping wound with some improvised sort of bandage made out of a towel or a torn sheet. Most of the men, however, lay there as they had been picked up by the villagers in the abandoned trenches or under the hedges along the muddy river bank. The two doctors had not half finished their round before the new-comer had taken out of his pocket his morphia syringe, once again to prove itself more valuable than all surgical instruments put together. The village doctor raised his hands to heaven in a gesture of despair. He took his colleague into the sacristy, and opening a cupboard in the wall he pointed to a row of old-fashioned faience jars, labelled with names in Latin of a dozen useless drugs and ointments. No morphia, no chloroform, no ether, no anæsthetics whatsoever ; no iodine, no disinfectants, no dressing material of any kind! The cupboard contained all that had been saved, said the Mayor, from the wreckage of the chemist's shop struck by the very first shell that had fallen on the village, killing the chemist outright, and destroying all its scanty supplies.

"I am not a surgeon," said the old village Doctor humbly. "I have never been a surgeon; all our surgical cases were sent to St. ——, and my other colleague here was mobilized as soon as the war broke out. I have no instruments, not even an artery forceps, and I should not know how to use them if I had any. Do you hear their groans? For three days and nights this terrible sound has not been out of my ears! It may be easier to bear for a young man like you— I am sure you are not half my age—but I feel I can stand it no longer, it is killing me. I am sixty-five, but I had hardly a grey hair three days ago. Look at me now; my wife says I am all white!"

The young doctor looked at the kind face of his old colleague, wondering to himself whether he would not rather have been one of the men on the straw-covered floor than to have had to live through these three nights and days as their doctor, powerless to help his patients to live, powerless to help them to die. And no morphia, priceless and mysterious gift from benevolent Mother Earth, giving power to the physician to bring relief to those the surgeon cannot help, to those who lie waiting for the other, the Great Physician who goes from bed to bed with his one remedy, his everlasting sleeping-draught!

"Listen to them," said the old Doctor, as if reading his colleague's thoughts, "and not even to be able to give them an injection of morphia!"

The other sat silent for awhile. "I am, alas! not more of a surgeon than you are," said he at last, "but we both know that surgery can do nothing for these dying men."

A hunchback, with quick restless eyes in an astute face ravaged by smallpox, entered the sacristy.

"Pierre started before daybreak, Monsieur le Maire," said he, "his mother sewed your letter in his waistcoat-lining, and I made him repeat all your instructions twice over. He is as clever as he can be, and I am sure if he does not succeed nobody else will. He was to keep away from the high road and ford the river below the mill."

"Well done, Anatole," said the Mayor, "and may God help him to return safe. He is quick of foot, and he ought to be back tomorrow morning if all goes well. This is the third messenger I have sent to St. ——," he said, turning to his colleague, "to get assistance for the wounded, and to tell them of our terrible plight. We are almost without food, all eatables were requisitioned for the retreating troops, and every cart and horse was taken from us for the evacuation of the wounded. Thousands of them passed through our village. Those you saw in there had been left as dead. Once the Germans had succeeded in blowing up the bridge there would besides have been no possibility of getting them away. There were many more here three days ago, and in a day or two there will be none left. They are dying one after another and I can do nothing for them!"

A handsome middle-aged woman with a small black shawl over her shoulders stood at the door.

"There is not a drop more milk in the whole village," said she despairingly, pointing to the pitcher she was holding in her hand.

"Be sure at least to give what there is to our men and not to that young Boche," said Anatole fiercely. "The Boches feed on blood and not on milk, and, believe me, he won't die, your young Boche, no more than will the big Uhlan next to him, who looks at one as if he wanted to eat one alive! And that brute of an officer with his Iron Cross, who has been yelling for another blanket the whole morning, and who cursed the Sister when she told him that the one he had was taken from Monsieur le Curé's own bed—he won't die either! Do you know that he ordered the German soldier next to him to give him his greatcoat and actually crawled out of his bed and took it from him! Believe my word, they won't die, the Boches! It is only our soldiers who are dying one after another; and the Boches will all get well and come back and murder our wives and children!"

"Shame, Anatole," said Josephine; "Boche or no Boche, they are all the same to me, these poor dying men. None of them will ever harm you or anybody else, and you need have no fear that even a Boche would like to eat you," she added hotly, as she went back into the church.

"Be quiet, Anatole," said the Mayor severely, "I have told you over and over again to leave those poor wretches alone; they could not help being born Boches. Anatole is our village barber," said the Mayor turning to the new-comer; "he is not as hard-hearted as he tries to make out. He has been most useful to us during these terrible days. He is as strong as a horse though he does not look it, and he has carried down more wounded than any of us."

"And if you had not ordered me to carry

down that young Boche instead of . . ."

The Mayor stopped him short with an uneasy glance at the door.

"I told you to be quiet, and if you go on like that I shall get downright angry with you. You know I am very sorry for you; but Josephine is even worse off than you—try not to forget it. Her husband was killed at Charleroi," said the Mayor to the Doctor; "her only son passed with his battalion through our village last Sunday, and she had just time to say ' God bless you ' to him as he marched past her in the street. His battalion held the ridge up there for the whole day under a terrible shell-fire. In the night the Germans charged with the bayonet. Nearly the whole battalion was annihilated; but she does not know it. She stood the whole day and night in the porch of the church, anxiously looking in the faces of the wounded as they were brought in. She has now made up her mind that her boy was amongst those few who got away. Since then she has never left the church, and I do not know what we would have done without her. It is besides the best thing for her to keep working. Neither the Curé nor I have had the heart to tell her yet——"

"Won't you come and look at him, Monsieur le Maire," pleaded Josephine at the door; "he is so pale, and his hands are so cold."

They all went back into the church.

The Curé was giving the last Sacrament to an officer who lay there motionless and silent, with half-closed eyes.

"He has never moved or spoken since he was brought here," said the nun, "but a moment ago as I wiped the perspiration off his face he said 'Thank you,' and turned his head towards the high-altar."

"Yes," said the other nun softly, "one can see by the way they are lying if they are conscious or not. All those who are conscious have their faces turned towards Our Lord."

"Water! Water!" murmured a soldier close by, who, as he lay there, with his face turned away, seemed to belie the nun's gentle observation. The soldier took the cup out of the nun's hand, and as he tried to put it to his lips it all dripped down his beard.

"He always wants to hold the cup himself," said she; "he does not seem to know that he is quite blind."

* *

"I am sure he is conscious and hears all we say," said the Mayor, stopping before another soldier. "Of course you may stay with him, but you must promise to sit quite still and not to talk to him, and above all you must not try to make him speak or he might spit blood again. And be sure the child does not disturb him," he added, pointing to the little girl sitting on the straw mattress at her father's feet. " I think you had better put her on the floor."

The little girl sat quite still, playing with a doll Josephine had just made for her out of a towel and some straw.

" Do let her stay," pleaded the wife, " she never leaves her father's side when he is at home, and I am sure he likes to have her on his bed. She is only four, but she understands everything, and she knows quite well she must not speak or make any noise. She has not uttered a sound since she crept on to his bed."

" Papa is asleep, you must sit quite still and not speak ! " whispered the child to her doll, putting her little fingers to her lips as she had seen her mother do.

" Perhaps you could persuade him to drink a little milk," said Josephine, as they bent over the soldier; " he has only had a drop of water since yesterday. And look ! " said she, gently lifting a corner of the greatcoat, " we have changed his straw twice since yesterday and now there is no more straw left in the whole village."

The unbuttoned tunic was soaked with fresh blood oozing from a terrible shrapnel wound in the chest.

"The gentleman is a doctor," said Josephine, covering the wound with a clean towel which slowly turned red as she spoke.

"Monsieur le Docteur, shall I soon get well?" murmured the soldier.

The Doctor watched his heaving chest and his superficial, irregular breathing, and said:

"Yes, soon."

"He is only twenty-five," said Josephine, "he is a *luthier*."

"A *luthier*! A violin-maker!"

"I never thought he would live through the night," said the Mayor in a low voice to his colleague. "But I must say that if anything his pulse seems to me a little better this morning, and I do think he is losing less blood. If only his heart can hold out."

"She is the image of her father," said Josephine, gently stroking the little girl's fair hair.

"Do you think so, Josephine?" said the wife. "I think the boy is much more like his father," she said, tenderly resting her tear-filled eyes on the rosy baby asleep on her lap. "If you knew what a wonderful child he is, Josephine! He never frets or cries, and nothing seems to upset him. I thought I was going crazy with the terrible roaring of the guns which has never ceased round our village for days and nights, but he did not mind it in the least. And did you ever see such a big boy, and so fat and firm! I am sure he will be as tall as his father. You know he was born only the day after the mobilization and his father has not seen him till now. I wish the doctor had let me put him on the bed for his father to have a real look at him, but the doctor said I was not to do it. I am sure he would not have cried; he never cries, and I am quite certain he knows it is his father, for he kept looking at him off and on before he went to sleep. I thought his father smiled at him a moment ago, but I am not quite sure. He looks at us the whole time, but now and then it seems as if he could not see us," she said, trying to keep back her sobs.

"I am sure he has seen the boy," said Josephine; "it is only that he is too tired to speak."

"Yes, I know," said the wife, "but if I only could be sure that he had seen the boy!"

"He must have lost an enormous quantity of blood," said the Doctor to his colleague, "his pulse is so very thin. I wish we could try to improvise some sort of transfusion apparatus to inject a warm saline solution into his veins. Do put another hot water bottle to his feet, Josephine; they are quite cold."

"Don't you think he is breathing a little better?" said the Mayor in a low voice. "Perhaps he is going to sleep."

"Perhaps," said the other.

The two doctors stood watching the soldier for awhile in silence.

Suddenly the little girl dropped her doll and looked up with terror-stricken eyes, her whole body trembling with fear and her face twitching with the effort not to cry.

"What is it?" said Josephine, looking uneasily at the little girl, "her face is quite white! Something has frightened the child!"

At the same instant the baby on his mother's knee started in his sleep with a sharp cry of distress.

The mother looked anxiously at her son and began to rock him to and fro in her strong arms.

"Something has frightened the boy . . ." said she.

The little girl flung herself from her father's bed and sprang to hide her face in her mother's lap.

"What is it?" said the old Doctor.

"I don't know," said Josephine, quite pale in the face, "I don't understand. Something has frightened the children!"

The soldier lay there just as before, his wide-open eyes looking towards his wife and child. The Doctor bent rapidly over him to listen to the heart, and made a sign to his colleague as he lifted his head.

"I would never have believed it," said the village Doctor, "it is hardly a minute since he spoke! I was looking at him the whole time and I did not notice anything."

"Neither did I," said the other. "It is very strange, but I have seen it once before. Small children know."

Josephine lifted the little girl in her arms, gently stroking her hair.

"Papa is asleep," whispered the little girl, putting her fingers to her lips and stretching out her other hand for the doll.

The soldier's wife opened her blouse and the boy began eagerly to drink life in deep draughts at his mother's breast.

* *

"Who is that?" exclaimed the Doctor.

The soldier was lying with his face towards the wall, and the broad collar of his khaki-coloured greatcoat turned up over his ears.

"I am so sorry," said the Mayor, "I quite forgot to tell you about him. He is an Englishman. We found him down by the river half buried under the wreckage of the blown-up bridge. The poor fellow was quite stunned. He has two of his fingers blown away, and he has a bullet wound in the back."

"Rather an unusual place for an Englishman to be hit in," said the Doctor.

"I have not been able to examine the wound very well, he is so very sensitive, and he begins to groan as soon as one touches him. He has had no internal hæmorrhage, and to-day his temperature is normal. His appetite is very good, he sleeps a lot, and I think he is doing very well considering."

"It takes a lot to kill an Englishman," said the Doctor.

"He does not speak French and none of us here understand his English, but we are trying to look after him as well as we can. You know we all like the English here," said the Mayor. "He will be very glad to see you."

"Hallo!" said the Doctor in English. "How are you getting on, Tommy Atkins?"

The man did not move.

"I think he is sound asleep," said the Mayor.

"His breathing is perfect, I do not think we need have any great anxiety about him," said the Doctor smilingly. "It does one's ears good to hear that snoring. I think the best thing we can do is to let him have his nap. I will come back to him by and by."

"He has a marvellous appetite," said the Mayor, "and is always ready for a glass of wine, and has no objection to a drop of brandy either."

"I quite believe you," said the Doctor, "but the fine thing about Tommy is that he is just as cheerful when he doesn't get it."

"He has just eaten a whole pot of marmalade," said the nun.

"I wonder how he came here," said the Doctor; "it is nearly thirty kilometres as the crow flies to the English line, but there are stragglers about everywhere."

"As far as I could gather," said the Mayor, "from something he muttered in, if you allow me to say so, most shocking French, he had been taken prisoner by the Boches and had managed to escape."

"Well done, and good luck for him that he fell in with your troops. Tell me when he wakes up," said the Doctor to the nun.

* *

They bent over another who looked at them with the terror of death in his deep-sunk eyes.

"Do you think she will come to-day?" he whispered to Josephine.

"It is his wife he is waiting for," said she softly; "he knows quite well he is dying, he has dictated two telegrams to her to come, and nobody has had the heart to tell him that all the wires are cut and no message can be sent anywhere with the Germans swarming all round us. I am sure she will come," said she, gently stroking his hand.

"Have you been a nurse before?" said the Doctor, "you are so patient and helpful to these poor men."

"No," said she simply, "but you see, Monsieur le Docteur, my boy is at the Front and I try to say to myself that if I am patient and kind to these poor fellows somebody else will be kind to him if he gets wounded. *Ah! le sang, le sang! Que Dieu punisse celui qui fait couler tant de sang!*" she suddenly cried out in terror pointing to a pool of blood on the floor. "It is not an hour since I washed it and there is the blood again!" She rushed to fetch a pail of water and began to wipe the marble floor.

The Curé looked at her with pitiful eyes.

"Her son is dead," he whispered to the Doctor; "we found his body up in the wood, and he was buried there with all the others. She does not know it yet."

They passed a long line of silent men with still white faces and half-closed eyes. They stopped before a big soldier with a rough bandage round his head and the blue cloak of the Saxon thrown over him.

"He has had no more convulsions," said the nun, "but he has never ceased to talk like this since this morning."

"He has a big hole in his skull from the splinter of a shell and has Jacksonian epilepsy," explained the old Doctor, "it is a marvel he is still alive. I am sure he ought to be trepanned, but how can we do it!"

The man's voice was still quite strong and he was talking with vertiginous rapidity. Dr. Martin bent over the Saxon, listening attentively to his incoherent flow of words; he put his hand firmly on the man's forehead and said, very slowly and distinctly, some words in German. The effect of the sound of his voice was instantaneous. The flow of words ceased at once and the man lay there motionless and silent as if listening to a voice from afar. After a moment he began talking again, and again he stopped as soon as the sound of words in his own language caught his ear. The Doctor sat quite still with his hand on his forehead, slowly and distinctly repeating the same words of greeting from the land of his birth. The intervals of listening silence grew longer and longer. His wild eyes gradually became steadier and his whole face twitched under a tremendous effort to regain consciousness. After a while he lay there quite still, looking fixedly at the stranger at his side.

"Where am I?" he murmured at last.

"With friends," answered the Doctor, fearless of his lie.

"Fritz?" said the Saxon hesitatingly.

"You are wounded, but you are with friends and you will soon get well and return home if you lie quite still and try to sleep."

"Yes," said he, and closed his eyes.

"Is he asleep?" said Josephine softly after awhile.

"No," said the Doctor, lifting his hand from the Saxon's forehead. "He is dead."

* *

"I am afraid he is very bad," said Josephine. "Monsieur le Maire says he is quite unconscious, he is bleeding internally and he has both his hands shot away by a shell.

He has never opened his eyes and never uttered a word since he came. He belongs to the same battalion as my son and they are great friends. Jean always goes to see him when he has any time to spare; their farm is only an hour from here. I always want Jean to be with him, he is such a nice quiet fellow; and he is such a wonderful gardener. He is their only son," said she, pointing to the two old peasant-folk sitting beside him. "I sent word to them that he was here and they came yesterday. They have been sitting here ever since. They do not seem to understand how bad he is. I have tried to make them see it and Monsieur le Maire has told them that he is very dangerously wounded, but it is quite useless, they don't seem to understand. Perhaps you could tell them; maybe it will have more effect if you say it."

"Yes," said the Doctor, looking attentively at the soldier, "they had better be told, it is high time. I have, alas! had to tell the same thing so often, and, if you cannot, I shall have to tell it again to these two."

The old farmer in his long blouse, his big horny hands leaning on his stick, sat looking with dim eyes at his son. The old woman in her neat white *coiffe* sat with her hands crossed over the basket on her lap.

"Monsieur is the new doctor," said Josephine.

The mother stood up and curtsied and the father raised his hand towards his head as if to take off his *béret*.

"I am so sorry for you," began the Doctor . . .

"Thank you, Monsieur le Docteur," said the old mother, "he has been asleep ever since we came, and I know well that is the very best thing he can do. He was always such a delicate child; I nursed him through all sorts of illnesses and I always knew that once he had gone to sleep he would wake up much the better for it. And don't you remember, père, when he fell down from the pear-tree and the doctor thought he had broken his skull, how he went straight off to sleep, and when he woke up he was out of danger? We do not mind sitting here the whole day; I have so often been sitting watching him sleep for hours and hours when he was a boy, and I say to his father to doze a little and that I will tell him as soon as the boy wakes up."

The old man blinked with his dim eyes approvingly, and leaned his chin against the stick.

"I wish he would just wake up for a moment to see that we are here, and then go off to sleep again. I am sure he wants to know all about the farm, and the vines, and the orchard, and his flowers. You know, Monsieur le Docteur, he was born on the farm and so was his father, and he has never left it. There is nobody like him for training vines, and whatever he plants grows like a miracle. It is only two years ago he made the new orchard, and the trees are already bearing—I have just brought this pear to show him. Look what a pear!" said she, producing a big Duchess pear out of her basket. " I am sure he will like to have a slice of it when he wakes up. And if you knew what a hand he is with flowers! There is not a farm anywhere like ours for flowers; even Madame la Comtesse when she drove past the other day said that in the Château itself there was not such a show of roses as we have. He has learnt it all by himself; he knows the names of all sorts of flowers, and those he does not know he himself gives names to. We did not mind the orchard, but we were a little against his turning the cabbage-land into flower-beds. We just want to tell him that we don't mind it any more, not even if he turns the whole kitchen-garden into flower-beds. We do not mind what he does, he is such a good and obedient son; the only disappointment he has ever given us was that he did not want to marry when his father wanted him to; he said there was not one girl in the whole country as pretty as his flowers, and that he liked better to keep company with them. The only quarrel he ever had with his father was when he wanted to go to work for a whole year under the head-gardener at the Château and become a real gardener himself. But how could we spare him on the farm, his father is getting so old! And now we want to tell him that he can become a real gardener if he wants. We will sell the cow and give him all the money he needs."

The old man scratched his head meditatively: "It is a very good cow, and don't you think we could see first what we could get for that old clock Madame la Comtesse always wants to buy?"

"He did not want to go to the war," the old mother went on, "but he said he must go. The last evening he took me out to his flowers and made me promise to look after them just as he had done, and he spoke about them as if they were alive. He always used to say that the flowers knew him and he never wanted to pick them, not even for the flower-show."

"Josephine, I think you had better tell

them," said the Doctor. "I don't know why, but I can't do it."

"Mère Christine," said Josephine, with her kind voice, "don't you understand that he is so dangerously wounded and has lost so much blood that he may never come back to you any more. He is so weak . . ."

"That is just what we have been talking about, le père and I," said the mother. "You know the Government has taken our horse, but we have thought that we would fetch him in the ox-cart, all filled with hay so as not to shake him. I know, Josephine, how good you have been to him, but don't you yourself think he would be better at home where he can lie out on sunny days in the garden amongst his flowers. It is so dark here," said she, looking round with awe. "His father was wounded in '70 and never got well in the hospital, but as soon as they took him home he began to get all right again. If only he wasn't so weak," said she, with an anxious look at her son, "but how can he be otherwise with not a morsel of food nor drink since he was shot, and all that blood ! If he only would wake up for a moment and eat something ! I just made this cheese for him before we left home," said the mother, taking a little cream cheese from her basket, "and I am sure he would like the pear . . ."

"Josephine," said the Doctor, "he is just dying."

* *

"Open the blinds, open the blinds! Why don't you open the blinds?" called out the soldier next to him. "Won't it be daylight soon? What o'clock is it? The night has been so long; won't you open the blinds?"

"These are the only words he says; he repeats them the whole time ever since he came," said Josephine.

"He has both his eyes blown in by a shell and both his legs torn away above the knee," explained the old Doctor.

"We also had a young officer here with his eyes blown in. We found him in a ditch beside the road; he looked quite dead, and it was only by his breathing that we understood he was alive. He remained quite dazed the first day, but yesterday morning he became conscious, and almost the first thing he did was to ask for a candle. It was broad daylight, so I knew he was blind. You could see nothing wrong with his eyes except that they were a little bloodshot. I put a bandage over them at once and told him they were inflamed, and that he must keep the bandage on for a day or two. He had at first some difficulty in articulating the words, but soon he began to speak quite well. He had not a scratch on his whole body, and only complained of a sharp pain in his head. He told me he was standing in the middle of the road when the shell passed close by him. He said the blast of air was as terrific as if an express train had dashed past him at arm's length, but a hundred times more so. He felt he was lifted from his feet and the tremendous displacement of air flung him in the ditch where we found him. He seemed to be doing so well that I really thought he was the only one here that was going to live. He asked several times to have the bandage taken away, as he couldn't stand the darkness. I said he must keep it on till to-morrow, to gain time to prepare him. We had so many to look after that it was impossible to watch him the whole time. A moment later Josephine came to tell me that he had torn off his bandage. After that he never uttered a word and he lay there quite still. When I came to look at him in the night I found he was dead . . . maybe better so for him!"

"Yes, better so for him!" said the other. "Better so for him!"

* *

"The Englishman is awake," reported the nun.

As the Doctor came up to him the man turned his head to the wall for another nap.

"Hallo, Tommy! How are you getting on?"

"Thank you, sir, very indifferently," said the soldier, without moving his head.

"Can I do anything for you?"

"No, thank you, I just want to sleep, that is all."

"I hope you don't suffer?"

"Awfully," said the soldier with a loud groan.

"You bear up well though; it is indeed lucky it doesn't affect your sleep. It did me good to hear you snore awhile ago. I am equally glad to know your appetite also remains satisfactory," said the Doctor, looking at the empty marmalade pot. "Don't you think we had better have a look at the wound in your back while you are awake, and try to cleanse it out for you. My colleague says it needs it badly."

"I am so weak," said Tommy, "and it

hurt me so much the last time that I don't think I can stand having it touched again."

"Suppose you have a drink first," suggested the Doctor.

"A drink?" said the soldier turning his head a little.

"I have still some whisky left in my flask, and you are very welcome to a drop of it."

The soldier stretched out his hand for the flask, his head still turned towards the wall.

"I am glad to see there is nothing wrong with your swallowing," said the Doctor, putting the flask back in his pocket. "Now tell me a little about yourself! What are you? I can't see anything of you but your greatcoat."

"Rifle Brigade," said the soldier.

"How on earth did you land here amongst the French? Where do you come from?"

"I don't remember the name of the place, I get so mixed up with the names."

"Menonville?" suggested the Doctor.

"That's the place," said the soldier.

"I have just come from there myself; rather a hot place, not very 'healthy,' as you Tommies call it. You will be glad to hear for your comrades' sake that they are soon going to clear out from there. I just happen to know that the whole Brigade is to take up another position."

"Where?" asked the soldier, with unexpected eagerness. "And the guns?"

"I do not remember, I get so mixed up with the names," said the Doctor. "I understand you were taken prisoner. How did that happen?"

"I was left alone in a trench with ten other men. We fought to the last, all the others were killed, and they took me prisoner, but I shot seven Boches first."

"Well done. Did you say seven?'

"Yes, seven."

"How did you escape?"

"I am so tired," complained the soldier, getting very feeble in the voice.

"Have a smoke," said the Doctor, taking a cigarette from his pocket. "It is true we are in a church, but smoking has now once for all been accepted in all ambulances, and I take the responsibility of letting you have a puff at a cigarette."

"No, thank you."

"Can't a Woodbine tempt you?"

"What?" asked the soldier.

"A Woodbine. You don't mean to say you don't know what a Woodbine is? If so you are the only man in His Majesty's Expeditionary Force who doesn't know it."

"I do not smoke," said the man.

"Don't you?" said the Doctor, his eyes

on the big burnt hole in the man's coat sleeve.

"What part of England do you come from?"

"I am a Canadian."

"Ah! that is where you get that slight American twang from. You were indeed lucky not to fall in with any Uhlans. They would have shot a khaki man at sight. There are lots of Uhlans about here. I had a hell of a time myself to get across from Menonville. Where did you meet the French?"

He did not answer.

"You are not very communicative; have another drink."

The Doctor bent over his face as he emptied the flask. "You need a shave badly," said he; "that hunchback standing over there is an excellent barber, and if you like I will tell him to give you a shave and a brush-up. You need it indeed. Your face is so covered with dirt and powder one can hardly see what you look like; one might take you for a minstrel on the beach at Margate. I know what you men like best, as soon as you are out of the fray and even while you are in it. And won't you be glad if I can manage to get you a cup of tea? I still have a small packet in my haversack."

"No thank you. I just want to sleep."

"All right. I see it is no good tempting you with anything; you want to be left in peace. You have deserved well of your country, and do have another nap, as that is what you want."

* *

"Won't you come and look at him, Monsieur le Docteur?" said Josephine; "he is so pale, and his hands are so cold."

They knelt down on each side of a young German soldier. His eyes were soft and light blue; his hair was curly and very blond, and the delicate moulding of his pale cheek was almost girlish. He looked barely eighteen.

"I am sure he is the same age as Jean," said Josephine. "I didn't know the Germans could look like this; he doesn't look as if he could do harm to anybody. I tried to give him a little milk, but I fear he cannot swallow," said she. "Do speak to him in German. I am sure he is conscious; he tried to say something, but alas! I can't understand his language."

A faint flush came to the boy's white cheek as he heard the first word in his own tongue whispered in his ear.

D

"Listen to me, but do not try to speak or you might spit blood again," said the Doctor. "We want to help you to get well and strong, and you will then return home again."

"Home?" whispered the boy.

"Yes, home—to your own home. Wouldn't you like to write home as soon as you are a little stronger? You will tell me what to say and I will write the letter for you and send it off. Perhaps we can write it tomorrow."

There came almost a smile on the lips of the boy.

"Now," he whispered.

"No, I think we had better wait till tomorrow."

"Now," he whispered again.

The doctor looked at him attentively and saw he was right. Josephine rushed to fetch a pen and paper in the sacristy, and in an almost inaudible whisper the boy began:

"*Meine liebe Mutter . . . !*"

Josephine's big shining mother's eyes filled with tears, for they had understood what her ears did not.

"*Meine . . . liebe . . . Mutter . . . !*" whispered the boy once again with still fainter voice. A slight shiver passed over him. His head turned towards Josephine, and it was all over.

" I wish I knew his Christian name ! " said Josephine, wiping her eyes.

* *

Two big bloodshot eyes had never left off watching the Doctor while he was busy with the dying boy. The eyes were all one could see of the man lying next to the boy ; his whole head was a big bundle of blood-stained towels and rough bandages, and his gigantic body was covered by the long cloak of a Bavarian soldier. The nun brought the Doctor some linen, torn off a sheet to replace the bandage dripping with blood. He almost wished he had not attempted it. The whole face and throat was one enormous wound: the jaw had been shot away and the tongue was torn. A sinister rattle accompanied his short and irregular breathing. All their efforts to give him some food or drink had failed, said the nun, and not even a drop of water had they succeeded in making him swallow. They cleansed his frightful wound as well as they could ; tried to remove the clots of blood obstructing the air passages, and raised his head to make him breathe a little more easily. With infinite trouble they succeeded, with the help of the village Doctor, in improvising a sort of tube through which they gave him a little wine and water. He was quite conscious, and maybe had been so ever since he was struck by the shrapnel. His eyes implored help. The Doctor sat at his side, feeling as though he almost wanted to beg his pardon for being so helpless. And he did it. He spoke slowly and as distinctly as he could, and he saw that the eyes understood his words. He said that they would soon get him a better bandage and a proper tube to feed him with. He told him he would then feel much better, and he promised to help him to get some sleep. He would soon feel stronger and breathe more easily, and he would soon begin to get well again. He spoke to the giant almost as one would speak to a child, slowly repeating the same words again and again:

"You will soon feel better, much better, you are so tired; you will soon feel better, your eyes are so tired, tired, your eyelids are feeling so heavy, so heavy, you are so sleepy, your eyes are closing, closing . . .

"Close your eyes!" said the Doctor, touching the eyes with his fingers. "Close your eyes!"

The unequal struggle between the strong, sound will and the exhausted brain tortured by pain lasted only a minute or two. The eyelids remained closed, the breathing became gradually deeper and more regular, and the restless hands lay there quite still.

The nun looked on in silent wonder.

"It is the first sleep he has had since he came," said she.

The Doctor sat at his side for a long while, not daring to move lest he should wake him. Josephine had come back, and he sat there watching her busy at work with the dead boy.

She washed his body clean from blood and mud and put a clean sheet under him. She dressed him in one of her own son's shirts she had evidently gone home to fetch; put a crucifix in his joined hands; lit a candle at the foot of his bed and laid a little bunch of flowers at his head.

"I am sure his mother would like me to do it," explained Josephine.

II

" I wish you had been here the first day to help us with the German major," said the Mayor. " You evidently know how to handle the Boches better than we do ; it seems as if you could do whatever you liked with them. I fear though that even you would have had some difficulty in tackling him. I ought not to say anything against him ; he is a dying man if he is not already dead, but I must say he was rather troublesome. He was shot through the shoulder, and I fear he was in great pain ; but he certainly was one of the least badly wounded here. He did not speak French very fluently, but he could quite well say anything he wanted. He was first lying next to the blind French soldier you have just seen ; but he complained that he disturbed him, and it is true that the poor man never ceases night or day calling to have the blinds opened. So we moved the major to the corner over there next to his own men. An hour later Sœur Marthe came to say that he was very angry and excited, and that he wanted to speak to me. I knew he was in pain, and I told him I was very sorry I could not do more for him ; and I begged him not to think it was because he was a German he was left in that state, but that, alas ! all the wounded were in the same terrible plight. Pointing to his Iron Cross he said it was an outrageous shame to neglect an officer like that, and that he must have an injection of morphia at once. I told him again that we had no morphia and that I had sent a messenger to St. —— for medicine and dressing-material, and I hoped surely to have some morphia for to-night, but that he must try to be patient till then. Sœur Marthe brought him a *tisane* of camomile—it was the only thing we had—but he threw it on the floor and said he must have morphia at once, and began to abuse us all first in French and then, as he grew more and more excited, in what sounded the vilest German. I might have told him that after all it was a German shell that had wrecked the chemist's shop ; but I said nothing. I did not know what more to say, so I left him, and told the nun to try again by and by with the *tisane*. So far he was in the right in a certain measure ; we all knew he was in pain and nobody minded his abusing us. But you could never guess the reason why he sent for me again in less than half an hour. When Sœur Marthe told it me I said she had misunderstood what he meant, and I had to hear it with my own ears before I could believe it. Do you know what he shouted as soon as I came up to him? He said he was a superior officer and that he must have a room to himself, and could not lie mixed up with his own men. His voice trembled with rage, and he worked himself into such a state of fury that he could no longer find words in French. Pointing to the German soldiers next to him he shouted the whole time a word in German which I did not understand; but I fear it was not complimentary, for I noticed that the soldier next to him looked at him angrily. This man is not mortally wounded either and is quite conscious, and speaks good French. He has an intelligent and rather refined face, and is, I believe, an educated man. He told me he was from Southern Germany, and that he was a Socialist and hated the war. Considering the state of excitement in which I had left the major, I was not very much surprised when Sœur Marthe came to report a little later that he had convulsions, and I admit I thought at first that his rage had ended in a sort of *crise de nerfs*. It was only in the afternoon that I began to suspect, from the stiffness of the throat, the fixedness of the jaws, and the increasing difficulty in swallowing, that the poor man had tetanus.

I have never seen a case of lock-jaw before, but I knew of course that he had to be isolated, and as we had nowhere else to put him we had to carry him into the charnel house. He indeed had tetanus, and tetanus in its most acute and violent form. In the evening he began having the most terrific attacks of tonic spasms, and the attacks have been increasing in intensity ever since. I need not tell you I have no serum, and even if I had I am sure it would be too late in his case. If I only had some chloroform, or ether, or morphia to help him a little in his worst attacks! All I could do was to darken the room and put straw on the floor to deaden the sound of our steps, as I have read that even a light or a sudden sound can, by reflex action, bring on an attack.

Early yesterday morning the South German trooper next to him began to show the same signs that had aroused my suspicions with the major, and we had to carry him also to the charnel house. The trooper, however, has so far only had some localized cramps in the jaw, and I have the impression that his case is much less severe. Nobody here has, of course, ever seen a case of this fearful illness, and it is difficult to make anybody stay with them. Sœur Marthe is there now and I have promised to relieve her at

Ave Maria. The bells will ring in a few minutes and I must go there.

"What a frightful disease!" he went on, as they walked across the cemetery; "and that they generally remain conscious to the very end makes it even more terrible to witness."

The place was quite dark but for the dim little oil lamp on the floor behind the heads of the two men who lay on each side of the room. The nun stood as near the door as she could.

"I am so afraid in this darkness," she whispered. "They are both quite still now; I had not heard the officer breathe for awhile," said she, "and I thought he must be dead. I read two Pater Nosters and it gave me strength to take the lamp and go up to him to put the crucifix in his hands. As I bent over him I looked at his face, and . . ." she burst into tears and put her hands before her eyes, "look at him!" she whispered with awe, "look at him!"

The Mayor took the lamp, and as the light fell on the dead officer's face he drew back in terror. The head was bent backwards in a last violent spasm, and the rigid muscles of the face stood still in a hideous laugh.

"*Risus sardonicus!*" said the Doctor.

"I have read about it in books, but I have

never seen it before, and I hope I shall never see it again!" said the Mayor, wiping the cold perspiration from his forehead.

"Is he dead?" asked the soldier from the other side of the room.

"Yes, I am afraid he is dead," said the Mayor, endeavouring to steady his voice. "It is no good trying to hide it from you. We had no hope about him from the beginning; but your case is quite different, and you will get all right if only you try to be calm, lie still, and do not speak."

"I am glad he is dead," said the soldier. "He commanded my squadron; I have lived in fear of him night and day for these two months. He has kicked me many times, and the last time he struck me with his whip across the face was the day before I was wounded. I am glad he is dead; it is no fault of his if there are still any of his men left alive, but if there are any I should like to live to be able to tell it them!"

"You must not speak," said the Doctor; "it is necessary that you should lie quite still and silent if you are to get well."

"You say it does me harm to speak; I say it does me good. I am going to have my say this time, they cannot stifle my voice any longer; I am a free man at last. You had better listen; it is the last speech of a German

Socialist that you are going to hear. My companions are silent, so far, but the day will come when they also will speak out, and with a far stronger voice than mine. I thank you for what you have done for me; it is not much, but I suppose it is all you could do. I heard you say to him that we wounded were better off on our side. Maybe it is so once we are in the ambulances, but before we are there we are worse off than on your side, for with us they pick up the officers first and leave us to the last. Did you hear what he called us when he told you he would not lie next to his own men? He could not find the right word in French in the fury he was in, but he found it all right in his own language. He called us *Schweine*, swine—that is how a Prussian officer speaks to his men! We obey them, cowards as we are, because we fear them; but we hate them as much as we fear them. —Yes, he called us swine, and he was quite right, and we ought to be grateful that he did not call us worse names. He might have called us thieves and murderers, and he would still have been right. Two months ago I was an honest man; I had not willingly offended either the laws of God or man, and I could look my wife straight in the eyes without fear or shame. Now I am a thief, a murderer, and a villain. I know I am damned, I know where I am going to, and I know who has led the way. It was he who led us through the burning streets of Louvain and through the smoking ruins of what was once called Aerschot; it was a peaceful town when we entered it and it was a blazing furnace when we left it. It was he who made us shoot the women and children at Dinant, and sprinkle their houses with petroleum and light them with our torches. It was he who made us loot and plunder Termonde and, drunk with wine and blood and lust, break into their houses and outrage their women. I rolled off to sleep that night with a bottle of champagne in my hand on the steps of the high-altar in one of their churches . . . so you had better spare your priest coming to see me through! Do not trouble about me, you Red Cross people, for I have shot lots of your wounded at Tamines! Don't read any Pater Nosters for me you, Sister, for I raped one of the nuns of the Sacré Cœur, whose prayers did not help her more than your prayers can help me. Well may you lie there and laugh at me, Major von Decken, for having been such a cowardly fool as to obey you so long. You were no coward—you! You were as brave as a man can be, but you were as cruel as a man can be: cruel to us, cruel to your enemies, cruel like the man-eating tiger! They say you can harm no more. I am not so sure of that; you had better not go too near him lest he might strike again. I have seen him laugh like that before. I know what that laugh means. It means that somebody is going to die."

The man's whole body stiffened in a frightful spasm, but his eyes remained lucid and calm, and the attack was soon over.

"Well, maybe it is only I who am going to die this time," he went on in a fearful voice. "Your impassible eyes will have to witness for once the death of a guilty man."

He lay silent for awhile, looking straight at his officer.

"But maybe it was not you alone who led us on; maybe you, too, brave as you were, lived in fear of somebody, somebody more strong, more cruel even than you! Maybe you were only the tool in a stronger hand than yours, as we were the blood-dripping tools in your hands. Whose hand was it? Colonels, Generals, Field-Marshals, Princes, Kings, and You! Emperor! To hell with you all for what you have made us do! You are sending me there now—I know it well—as you have sent thousands of your men there before. I die without fear, for death can have no new terror to spring upon me that life has not revealed to me during these last months. I am not afraid of hell, for no tortures the devil ever inflicted upon the damned can be more terrible than the torments you, with the name of God on your lips, made us inflict upon righteous men and harmless women and children—in fact you have added to the list ; you have proved a first-rate expert in inventing instruments of torture—the devil will have a lot to learn from you !

" You willed the war, sinister Emperor ! You wanted to become the world's greatest ruler ; you have become its greatest criminal. The sun is setting blood-red and menacing over the tottering walls of your world-power ; your short day of triumph is drawing to its close, your long night of expiation is about to begin. I have seen your restless eye—the fear of death is already there. But better no gallows for you ! Better to suffer you to live on with that fear in your eye ! Better to let you die in your bed assisted by your acquiescent Court-Chaplains trying in vain to silence your cry of anguish with their litanies, and surrounded by your bowing Court doctors working their hardest for you to hold on a few hours longer to your dishonoured crown and to rouse you from the invading torpor that you may hear to your very last breath the maledictions of your victims.

"You are fond of travelling in pomp. Better to let you start in state for your last show, your last journey, to the sound of merry chimes from all the ruined belfries of Flanders and the bells of Rheims calling France to Mass to offer thanks to God! Better to let you go to hell with all the honours due to your rank as the greatest slayer of life, the greatest destroyer of happiness the world has ever known!

"We who are going before you to our doom—we shall all be there to welcome you, to close round you as your bodyguard, ready to die for our Emperor once more if ever heaven would dare to storm hell to try to reconquer your soul!

"Do you hear the clatter of their horses' hoofs? Do you see their lance-tips glistening in the dark? They are coming, they are coming! Hurrah! It is my squadron—it is the Death's Head Hussars! It is all my dead comrades riding to hell! Help me to the saddle!"

The bells began to ring Ave Maria. As the sound struck his ears his hands instinctively made the sign of the Cross. His jaw closed, his whole body grew rigid with a terrific spasm, and the heart stood still.

III

"This beats anything I have ever seen or heard," said the old village Doctor as they walked across the churchyard. "And this last rigid spasm of the muscles of laughter, this hideous *risus sardonicus*, do you mean to say it often occurs in tetanus?"

"Often enough," said the other, "I have seen it several times. There have been, as you know, an appalling number of cases of tetanus, both with the English and the French. I am sorry that this man is dead, I wish he had been spared to his country, a dozen Socialists as far gone as he are worth a whole brigade for breaking down the stronghold of Prussian militarism. Did you see the glare in his eye when he started cursing the War Lord? If, as he said, they are to meet in another world, no doubt he will see to it that the Kaiser gets a warm reception on his arrival in that place. I wonder who he was; for all we know he may have been one of the leaders of his party; his flowery and rather theatrical way of speaking points to his being accustomed to address a larger audience than he had to-day."

"I shall never go back to that charnel-house again," said the old Doctor, "not even Balzac could have conjured up a more ghastly scene."

"It makes me think of Dostoievsky," said the other. "It is just what he would have liked. But fiction is indeed a tame business compared to reality, and Life is, after all, the most daring and the most original writer of startling tales the world has ever produced. Your Balzac was a great reader of medical handbooks, and so was Dostoievsky, and no doubt they could have described such a death scene—*risus sardonicus* and all—accurately enough. But would either of these great masters have dared to put in the mouth of their dying German soldier that long harangue about the Emperor? I doubt it. They would have thought it far too melodramatic to be true to life. Why is it that people in a semi-delirious state not infrequently speak with a wealth of ideas and an exuberance of imagery which often makes them quite eloquent? Mad people are often most brilliant and witty in their conversation, and as to their power of argument . . ."

"The sharpest lawyer I ever heard of was a lunatic, and nobody thought anything of him as long as his mind was sound," said the old Doctor.

"The Englishman is awake," reported Sœur Philippine at the door of the church.

"I am delighted to hear it," said Doctor Martin. "We are both in need of a little diversion, my dear colleague; I want to have another talk with that Englishman of yours, and I would like you to be present at our conversation."

"He knows no more French than I do English," said the Mayor, "so I shouldn't understand a word."

"I think you will understand this time."

"I hope he did not complain and that you told him how sorry we are not to have been able to do more for him. We all like the English so much. We had lots of them billeted in our village last month when the English were holding the line here. They used to give the children chocolates and jam, and carry them on their shoulders and play all sorts of games with them, whenever they were not drinking tea or washing themselves under the pump, which they did most of the day. They paid almost double its value for everything they took, and always thought first of the welfare and comfort of their horses and then of their own. All our women-folk were crazy about them, and no wonder, for a smarter-looking set of men I never saw, all tall, clean-looking chaps, and so merry. They were always laughing, several of them were wounded, and not slightly, but they hobbled about laughing just the same. They didn't speak a word of French, no more than this one does in the church, but it was extraordinary to see how they got on with the children; they understood each other quite well. Anatole also says he understood them, but I am not so sure about that. He says he had never had such a time in his life—they always wanted shaving. They were here over a Sunday, and lots of them came to church, and the Curé delivered a special sermon for them, and he said he had never had a more sympathetic or responsive congregation, although they evidently did not understand a word he said. The others held divine service on the Green; one of their officers read a short sermon and all the men sang a hymn and knelt for their prayers, and I must say it was most impressive."

"Did you look at this one's face?" asked the Doctor.

"Yes, yes . . . we all like the English over here."

As they came up to the Englishman Anatole was just helping him to a glass of wine, with some friendly remarks in an unknown tongue constructed out of his previous dealings with his friends *les Anglais*.

" I love the English," said Anatole, " but somehow I do not get on as well with this one as I did with the others; they spoke better French than he does."

" I am not so sure of that," said the Doctor, " I think it is only that he is rather shy. Don't be so shy, Tommy," he continued in French, turning to the soldier. " Surely you don't want to disappoint your kind friends here by forcing me to carry on our little conversation in a language they don't understand. We know you were somewhat stunned when the bridge was blown up; maybe it is that which made you forget your French. Now that your head is quite clear again you will see it will all come back to you quite nicely. But do pull down that collar of your greatcoat, so that we may look at your face while we talk; we all like the look of an Englishman who has killed seven Boches. Now tell me a little more of your glorious past; I don't expect you to tell the truth, but you might try. We will talk about the future by and by. Where did you pick up that excellent French of yours?" The man's eyes wandered restlessly round the church.

" He doesn't speak a word of French," explained Anatole.

" Answer ! " said the Doctor, his dark eyes rivetted upon the soldier.

The man looked uneasily from one to the other of those around him, till at last, with a quivering of his eyelids, he faced the doctor:

" It is all up," said he in perfect French.

" Answer ! " said the Doctor.

" I have been in Belgium these last two years."

" What became of you when the war broke out ? "

" I became dispatch-rider to the General Staff, but had to give it up on account of my weak heart."

" How long were you with the English ? "

" Since after Mons."

" In what capacity ? "

" I served first in the Transport service, and then as chauffeur with a Red Cross motor ambulance."

" You were then a Belgian refugee, I suppose ? "

" Yes."

" And you were an English straggler when you were with the French ? You did good work ? "

" I think so, for I was promoted."

" Who had you to report to ? "

" To my nearest superior, who was interpreter to the General Headquarters."

" You had no difficulties ? "

" No, it is easy with the English."

"More difficult with the French?"

"Yes, by far."

"I daresay your khaki uniform was very useful to you."

"Yes, rather."

"I have just been admiring your greatcoat, it almost looks like an officer's; you are a great swell! Did you kill your man, or did you rob the dead—hyena fashion?"

"All our khaki uniforms are made in Düsseldorf," said the man with a certain pride.

"Now my dear Fuchs, or Katz, or whatever may be your name—shall we call you Fuchs, it fits you nicely. Now my dear Fuchs, let us come to the little accident in your career which gave us the pleasure of your acquaintance."

The man groaned loudly.

"No, Fuchs, I wouldn't try that groan again if I were you; it brought you such bad luck last time you tried it. When a clever man like you, Fox, gets himself up as a Tommy he ought to know that an Englishman does not groan when the doctor dresses his wound; he never utters a sound, he clenches his teeth if it comes to the worst—but that is all. Nor would any self-respecting Tommy ever dream of growing that dirty red beard of yours; he would have had it shaved off, and had a wash long before he ate that pot of marmalade. You were quite right about that marmalade though, and you were also quite welcome to the drink considering the circumstances; but be careful, Fuchs, don't overdo it! You made an awful mess of it when you did not stretch out your dirty fingers for that Woodbine I offered you, and that you did not feel like a cup of tea was an equally bad shot, my poor Fuchs. I have yet to live to learn that there exists a Tommy who resists a Woodbine or a cup of tea. Your greatcoat was all right, but, my dear Fuchs, it was your head which got you into trouble, and you were quite right to duck it under your collar. Look, Anatole, at your friend Fuchs, you who know *les Anglais*, did you ever see an Englishman walk about with such a head?"

Anatole's eyes had become quite small, and crouching like a big cat ready to spring, he drew nearer and nearer to the spy.

"No, Anatole, not yet," said the Doctor. "We know, my dear Fox, that you are storing a French bullet somewhere in your anatomy which might have killed an honest man, but by some oversight of the devil did you but little harm. I have an uncomfortable sensation that you intended to take up your profession again in a very short time, and that you would in all probability have succeeded had I not had the advantage of meeting you here. Had the soldier who sent that bullet into your back discovered one minute before that there was a traitor among them, there would be no wounded in this church to-day. You had just time to light the fuse which blew up the bridge and your two fingers as well. You knew that it meant the lives of all those men whose bread you had shared and who no doubt had offered you their last cigarette, and whatever little comfort they may have had, as homage to the uniform you wore—you say it is all right so; it is what you call war, isn't it so, Fox?"

"It hurt my feelings to do it, but I had to carry out my instructions, and it nearly cost me my life."

"Did you say nearly?"

The man's face grew ashy grey under its layer of dirt.

"No, Fuchs, you needn't worry. We do not kill wounded men in an Ambulance, not even a wounded spy. I am sure you will be given ample time to collect your varied impressions of these last months. You have indeed shown yourself worthy of your promotion."

"If you spare my life I will give information to your authorities for which your Secret Service would pay a fortune."

"I am glad you told me this, Judas Fuchs; it was nice of you, it facilitates matters for me personally a lot. I have, like you, a sentimental nature; it hurts my feelings to cause a man to be shot and I was almost beginning to feel sorry for you, my dear Fuchs."

The spy succeeded in getting his eyes away from the Doctor's, and he cast a rapid glance at the door.

"Yes, you are quite right, Fox, the doors are left open the whole night; but you are wrong in thinking that you might wriggle out like a venomous reptile in the dark. Listen well to what I now tell you! You will never come out alive from this church. If man does not kill you, God will."

Fear shone in the eyes of the spy and his whole body began to shiver.

"Are you certain he won't escape?" said the Mayor as they turned away. "I have heard of a man with a bullet through his body being able to walk in less than a week's time. It may besides be true what Sœur Philippine told me, that she thought she saw a shadow moving last night towards the door. Who else could it have been but he? I dare not rely on anybody to watch him during the night. We are all worn out; we must keep the doors open, the stench is too terrible, and we have besides all the dead to carry out during the night. Who can guarantee that he does not crawl out through the window?"

"Why not put him in the charnel-house?" said Anatole. "It's the very place for him."

"No," said the Mayor, "I think we will not put him there; we will like it better so when our heads are cool."

"Quite so," said the Doctor, "and I take the responsibility before you, Monsieur le Maire, that he shall not escape. He is welcome to try; I know he cannot do it. I know I can hold him; he is not only a spy but he is also a coward, which is, I believe, a rare combination in his dangerous profession. I saw a spy shot a week ago, and I could not help admiring his courage to the very end. This scoundrel, who wanted to betray his own country after having already betrayed three other countries, is quite harmless now; he is shaking all over with terror, and he will die of fear if of nothing else.

"He is not fit to lie here amongst these brave men," said the Doctor as they walked down the nave. "I have felt ever since I entered your church as if service were going on the whole time, and there is something blasphemous in his being here. But I have a feeling that it won't be for long."

* *

"Did I show you the big Uhlan over there, *mon cher confrère*," said the old village Doctor pointing down the side aisle. "He was shot through the spine and I fear he suffers terribly. Luckily for him I believe the end is near; it looks to me as though he would not be here to-morrow."

"Yes, I know him well," answered his colleague, "he is the only Boche here who is able to speak; I had a long talk with him this morning; we are great friends. I do not know if he is a Uhlan or not; he is so covered with blood and mud that it is impossible to make out what his uniform is. All I know of him is that he took part in the massacres of Dinant."

"He looks like it," said the old Doctor. "We found him down on the river bank under some willows; he was almost lying in the water. He is the biggest man I ever set eyes on; Anatole says it was quite a job to lift him. He had a collapse when we took him from the stretcher and put him on the straw; in fact, I thought he was gone. As I bent over his face to see if he was dead he opened his eyes, and he startled us all with such a terrible scream that one could hear it all over the church. He screams whenever one comes near him. I never saw such a wild-looking man. They are all rather afraid of him here.

Anatole thought he was going to strike him when he wanted to lift him; he has the fists of a giant. Did you ever see such a ferocious face?"

"*Il n'est pas méchant*," said Josephine, who was standing behind the Uhlan so that he could not see her, "but he does not want anybody to look at him. I believe he is afraid of somebody."

"You are as clever as you are good, Josephine," said Doctor Martin; "you are quite right, he is afraid of somebody. It is nobody here."

"He has been following you with his eyes the whole time," said she. "Do talk to him; I am sure he is longing to speak to you."

"Thank God you have come back," said the Uhlan, as soon as he heard the Doctor's voice. "Did you see anybody as you came?" he added in a hurried whisper.

"No."

"Are you sure?"

"Quite sure."

"She always goes away when you come," he murmured.

"Who?"

He closed his eyes. "The old woman," he said with a shudder. "I was afraid you were not coming back."

"I promised you I would come back."

"Yes, but since I told you this morning about the old . . ." He closed his eyes again.

"I have forgotten all about her," said the Doctor.

"I want to tell you," the soldier went on with an unsteady voice. "As I bent over her face to see if she was dead . . ."

"I do not want to hear anything more about her," said the Doctor sternly; "you may tell me anything you like, but I do not want to hear anything more about the old woman."

He looked quite disappointed. "But you said you had forgotten. As I bent over her face to see if—for God's sake let me tell you," he pleaded eagerly, as the Doctor tried to stop him again, "for God sake let me tell you! I cannot bear it alone any longer, I feel as if you might help me if you knew all about her. I am sure you can help me; she went away when you spoke to me this morning; it is the only time she has left me since I came here. As I bent over her face to see if she was dead," he went on with unmistakable relief . . .

The Doctor saw he was powerless to spare the man his self-inflicted torture. Helpless and silent he sat by the soldier's side listening once more to the gruesome tale of the massacre of the eight hundred civilians at Dinant. He knew the terrible story through the depositions of the few survivors; he heard it now from the trembling lips of one of the executioners.

It was all carried out with order and precision; the officers were there to see that the work was properly done, and that it all went off without a hitch—the men were rather more drunk than was good for them. One of his comrades was shot dead by an officer as he threw down his rifle when orders were given to fire on the defenceless crowd. They slaughtered the men first, several hundreds of them, mostly old men, but many mere boys. Then the women by hundreds, mothers and wives, daughters and sisters, young and old. How many he had shot he did not know, he did not remember, nor did he seem to worry much about it. It was all about the old woman. He saw her running down the street, but she could not run very fast, she was a very old woman—" *Eine sehr alte Frau,*" said he. He stabbed her as she was entering a house; she fell on the threshold. As he bent over her face to see if she was dead, she opened her eyes and looked at him with the same eyes as his grandmother had looked at him the day he started for the war and bid her farewell in their village church—the same sad, humble eyes. The old woman was holding her prayer-book and her spectacle case in her hand, just as his grandmother was holding her prayer-book and her spectacle case in her old hands. She was quite dead, but she kept on looking at him.

He ran to join his comrades and they all sat down round the bonfire in the midst of the square to a hearty meal with an extra ration of sausage and potatoes, and many good things they had looted from the shops, and as much wine as they could drink, and all the dead bodies lying round them as they had fallen. The officers dined outside the café close by, and the tables were laden with champagne bottles—it was all very jolly, "*Sehr lustig*" he called it. The men sang "*Deutschland über Alles*," and at the end, "*Nun danket alle Gott*." He got quite drunk again and felt very happy. Just as he was dropping off to sleep that night the old woman came and bent over him and looked at him with the same eyes as his grandmother. Since that day she came regularly every night as he was going off to sleep and bent over him and looked at him, just as his grandmother used to come and look at him when he was a boy—for he had never known his mother. He stood it for a week, but then he got so exhausted from want of sleep that he could hardly walk, and he was reported to the doctor. The doctor gave him a pill which made the old woman come a little later at night and also in the day as soon as he was alone. Then he was put under arrest for something he had done he did not remember, and for two days and nights the old woman never left his side and kept looking at him the whole time. He then thought he would speak to the army chaplain. He was a very good chaplain— a God-fearing man much liked by all the men. The chaplain cured him on the spot. The chaplain said it all came from the stomach, that he had nothing to worry about, that he was defending the Fatherland, and that the old woman would probably have gouged out the eyes of one of his comrades had she lived—if she had not already done it. The kind chaplain managed to get him out of prison and the next day he was quite fit again, and never once did the old woman come back to look at him during their whole advance through Belgium and France. The night he was wounded she came back again and looked at him with his grandmother's eyes. He tried to crawl away from her and hide under some willows, but she followed him

F

there and for the whole day and night she kept on looking at him. He begged her for God's mercy to fetch him a drop of water from the river, but she never moved and never took her eyes off him. He did not know how many days and nights they remained there, but he remembered quite well that one of the men who came to carry him away on the stretcher was a hunchback. The night was dark, but he could see the old woman distinctly as she walked at the side of the stretcher, her white hair flowing in the wind and her clothes dripping with blood. As they carried him up the church steps the bells in the old village church began to chime their well-known chime, and at the door stood Hans, the old beadle, who used to chase him and the other boys away when they were too noisy during Mass; and Hans nodded to him as he passed. He saw his grandmother in her white cap and her black shawl kneeling on her old knees in her usual place by the side altar. He was not very surprised to see her there, for he knew she would come every evening to pray for him. He wanted to go up to her, but he thought he had better wait till she had finished her prayer. The old woman from Dinant was gone. He looked at his grandmother; he knew he was safe, he knew he was released, and he would have thanked God had he dared. As they lifted him out of the stretcher all the lights in the church went out, and it became dark as death around him. He had ceased to suffer, so he thought he had ceased to live. And again he wanted to thank God had he dared. A wild cry of distress woke him from death. It sounded far, far away, but he thought it was almost like his own voice.

He opened his eyes and he saw moving lights around him. He looked for his grandmother, but she was gone. He was lying on the straw-covered floor of another church, and around him were groans and shrieks and blood and dying men. He closed his eyes again. A shadow fell over him. The old woman from Dinant stood bending over him and looking at him. Since that day she had never left him; night and day she was there at his side.

"Did you see anybody as you came?" he whispered with a shudder. "For God's sake stay with me; she will come back if you go away. Don't go away; for God's sake stay with me!"

He lay there timidly fumbling about with his hand in search of the Doctor's, as if afraid he might not be allowed to hold on to his hand. He was sinking rapidly. His eyes were growing dim.

"Look!" said the Doctor, pointing down the side aisle towards the altar. "Look! your grandmother has come back! Look! she is there in her white cap and her black shawl kneeling on her old knees in her usual place!"

He raised his head eagerly and stared with his dim eyes towards the altar.

"It is getting so dark," said he, "I cannot see!"

"Look! she is lighting a candle to show you the way! Now she is kneeling again, don't call her! She is praying for you! Can't you see her now?"

He tried to raise his head once more. "The candle, the candle, yes, I see the candle, the . . . Grannie! Grannie!" he called almost with the voice of a child. "Grannie!" he whispered again quite gently, so as not to disturb her whilst she was praying.

He lay there silent for awhile, looking steadfastly at his grandmother. His wild features grew soft and still, and big tears rolled down his cheek.

He had not suffered enough. Once more the horror of the past gripped at his weary brain, once more he turned with fear-filled eyes towards the Doctor.

"Do you think I am going to hell?" he whispered with awe.

"No," said the other. "I believe God is listening to your grandmother's prayers and that He will have mercy on you and let you go to heaven."

He looked at his grandmother again. A few moments later the terror went out of his eye and such a peace fell over his anguished face that the Doctor believed he was right.

IV

THE old village Doctor, worn out by his long watch, had consented to let his young colleague take his place for the night, and Josephine had also been persuaded to go home for a little rest. The two nuns sat already huddled together in their usual place fingering their rosaries, and Anatole was to share the night watch with the Doctor and call the Curé in case of need. The Doctor had noticed that a mattress had been brought over from the Presbytery and placed in a corner of the sacristy, and he had seen Anne, the Curé's old cook, come and put bread, cheese, and grapes, and a flask of wine on the table under the ominous cupboard.

The nuns lit the candles on the altar and a couple of oil lamps in the side aisles. Kneeling before the Madonna's shrine Sœur Philippine read out the prayer for the night:

Priez pour nous pauvres pécheurs maintenant et à l'heure de notre mort!

It grew darker and darker in the church.

With a small oil lamp in his hand the Doctor went his round. Now and then a shrill shriek of pain or a deep sigh pierced the gloom, and terror spoke to him out of wide-open eyes, and the desperate grasp of a hand implored him for help.

Night came at last with its blessed hush of silence.

He bent over the white faces on the floor, and as often as not he did not know where this silence meant sleep and where it meant death.

Some of them looked as if they did not know it themselves, as if unaware that their sleep was the sleep of eternity. The *luthier* lay there with the crucifix in his hands, calm and serene as if listening to the vibrating voice of the beloved violin his long, delicate fingers had just moulded out of some piece of dumb wood. The other, who had been lying there for three days and nights staring out of his darkness for the sun to rise at last, now looked as if he could see better than anybody else, as if he saw straight into heaven. Close by lay Josephine's boy hero on his white sheet, immaculate from pollution and blood, immune from bullets and wounds, beautiful and flower-crowned like a young god!

"Where is the German officer who stole the greatcoat from the soldier next to him?" said the Doctor to the hunchback.

"I have not heard his cursed voice for

awhile," said Anatole, taking the oil lamp in his hand and leading the way to the side aisle. He lay there the last in the row close to the side entrance. His marble-white forehead was high and clear, his strong features were manly and bold, and his wide-open, still eyes looked straight and fearless at his accuser.

"I do not believe that story about the greatcoat," said the Doctor to Anatole.

* *

The two bloodshot eyes under the bundle of bandages opened as the Doctor bent over the Bavarian giant.

"Thank God you have had a little sleep! Now we are just going to cleanse your mouth and syringe your throat from all that nasty stuff which is choking you. If you lie very still whilst I do that you are going to have a drop of wine and water like last time—or would you rather have some milk?"

The nun whispered that there was none, but luckily the Bavarian had already chosen the wine and water, according to how the Doctor read his eyes.

"Wasn't I right that you preferred wine and water? There, you see that I can understand by your eyes what you want to say, so it is quite useless for you to try to speak, which is very bad for you. I understand you and you understand me, and that is all we want—isn't that so?"

The giant nodded, and his eyes twitched with the pain as he did so.

"Don't nod, I know you just wanted to say you are pleased you have found a man you can talk to like this, and if you are very patient and still while I put that tube down your throat, I will tell you what you and I are going to do to-morrow morning after you have had another snatch of sleep."

The eyes signalled that they wanted to know at once.

So the Doctor told him that they were going to help each other to write a letter home to tell his wife he was getting on quite well and would soon be home again. The giant nodded so that the whole bundle of bandages shook, and the eyes half closed with pain.

"I told you not to nod," said the Doctor as severely as he could, and the eyes begged pardon at once.

"Won't he suffer too much to have that hard tube down his throat again?" said the nun timidly.

"No, he will stand it much better this time, and he longs besides for a little water down his burning throat, and he badly needs a few drops of wine too. Try to get us some milk for to-morrow if you possibly can. That he is still alive means that he intends to make a hard fight, and he will let us do with him anything we want. He is as docile as a lamb, and he will go off to sleep again as soon as we have cleansed his throat and fed him a little."

"How can you make him go to sleep so peacefully?" said the wondering nun.

"I know no more than you how I can make him sleep, Sister, but I know that I can do it," said the Doctor gravely.

He had finished his round closely followed by the hunchback, who did not seem to want to leave his side for a minute. Overpowered by fatigue and almost faint from the terrible stench which rose like a deadly mist from the floor, the Doctor sat down on the bench near the entrance door looking into the starlit night for the dawn which seemed never to want to come.

"It does my eyes good to look at the stars," said he.

"Will this night never come to an end!" groaned the hunchback.

"What's the matter with you, Anatole?

You look quite ill, and you are shaking all over."

"Did you see how he stared at me? I can't get over those dead eyes!" said the hunchback, his voice trembling with fear.

"Why don't you go home for a couple of hours' sleep? There will be plenty to do for us all to-morrow, and I can manage quite well here with the two nuns."

"I dare not go out in that black night," said Anatole; "for God's sake let me stay with you till it gets light, if it ever will. I have, besides, nowhere to go to. Don't you know that my shop was knocked down by a shell, and my wife was killed on the spot?"

"No, my poor Anatole, I did not know, or I would not have told you to go home. Of course you stay with me; I am very glad to have you here. I don't feel, either, as if I wanted to be here alone."

In order to distract Anatole from his gloomy thoughts, the Doctor then began to ask about the last days' fighting around the village. Anatole told him how the battle had been raging all around them for several days, how during a whole afternoon shells had been falling over the village, how though outnumbered by five to one a battalion of their men had held the bridge-head for the whole day.

"When orders were given to retreat, the Boches had already succeeded in blowing up the bridge, and the whole battalion was massacred. Our troops made a last stand on the ridge of scattered pines up there overlooking the village; you can see there are hardly any trees left now, and the whole slope was thickly covered with wood before. At daybreak the Boches made a furious bayonet charge and there was a desperate hand to hand fight, but they were repulsed. At noon they began to shell the hill again until there was hardly one of our men left alive. Nobody in the village went to bed that night. We expected the Boches to come at any moment; but they never did, or I should not be here to tell the tale. They kill everything, women, children, and cripples. The next morning a wood-cutter came down and told us that the whole wood was full of dead lying in heaps one upon another, and that he had found a soldier still alive outside his hut. He had crawled there during the night, and he said he was sure there were others still living among the dead. We improvised some sort of stretchers, and I went up there at once with the Curé and the Doctor and the few old men still remaining in the village. During that day and the following night we carried down, I think, nearly two hundred men who the Doctor said were still alive, although most of them looked quite dead, and many were actually dead when we got them down here, and many have died since. I don't think there are more than about half of them here now. We also found several Boches alive. We wanted to carry down our men first, but both the Curé and the Mayor said we must take them in turn as we found them. I wish we had not done as we were told; if it had not been for that, poor Jean would not have been lying there now amongst all the dead Boches. I shall never dare to tell the truth to Josephine, for she will never forgive me. Jean's body was one of the last we found. It was I who found him with a bayonet thrust clean through his chest. When I came back to fetch his body the others had already buried him by mistake. The Mayor had said that all the dead must be buried the same night, and they had all been heaped together in the big abandoned trenches and earth shovelled over them. I shall never dare to tell Josephine the truth, for she will never forgive me. Maybe it is not so in your country, but with us our women folk want to know the spot where their sons are lying and want to put a cross and some flowers on their graves. And poor Josephine will never know where to put her flowers and where to pray, for the whole wood is full of dead, and there are all those Boches amongst them, and nobody knows where Jean lies. He was everything to her and he was so good to her. And if you knew what a fine lad he was, tall and strong like his father and with his mother's big brown eyes. She will never forgive me, I know she won't."

He sat silent awhile. His restless eyes kept wandering round the dark church and suddenly stood still, staring fixedly towards the corner where Josephine's candle was burning.

"Do you see that candle? Do you know who killed Jean?" he whispered suddenly.

"No," said the Doctor with unsteady voice.

"It was that young Boche she has been nursing night and day who killed her son," said he fiercely. "Jean was lying under a tree a little way from the others. The bayonet had entered his left side near the heart, and the point was sticking out under his right arm-pit. The Doctor said he must have been killed instantaneously. The Boche lay beside him in a pool of blood with both his hands still on the butt-end of his rifle. The Doctor said I must pull out the bayonet, but my hands shook so that I could not do it. The Doctor said he could not do it either, so I had to do it. As I took hold of the rifle the Boche grabbed at it, and we saw he was still alive. He had been shot through the chest the same instant he thrust his bayonet through poor Jean. The Doctor said the bullet had pierced both his lungs near the heart, and that he had lost so much blood that it was a marvel he was still alive. Both the Curé and the Doctor said it was not right or Christian to leave him there, so we were made to carry him down first, and when Pierre and I came back for Jean they had already buried him. I shall never dare to tell Josephine the truth, for she will never forgive me."

"Listen, Anatole," said the Doctor. "I see you are all right again and don't mind sitting alone for a few minutes. I just want to go outside the porch for a moment and smoke a cigarette. You remain sitting where you are and call me at once if somebody wants me."

He went out of the church and stood for a long while in the middle of the chaussée. He felt as if he could not understand, would not understand, and as if he wanted to ask for an explanation. He looked up to the stars that had explained to him so many riddles, but their cold glitter flashed no message to his dark thought. He looked towards the Eastern hills for some light to come to his anguished soul, but there was no sign of any dawn. Were they, then, all blind, those shining eyes overhead, or how could they look so indifferently on all the wounds, all the tears, and all the horror of the night? Was there, then, no pity in the sun that was soon again to purple yonder hills with blood, soon again to light the track for Death to stalk his victims from valley to valley, from cliff to cliff? What had this fair world done to be thus torn asunder by the sinister birds of prey of evil, what had these poor men done to be driven to murder those they were meant to love!

A sound of unspeakable terror came hissing through the poplars along the chaussée, splitting the darkness with lightning speed as it flew past him. A terrific blast of air lifted him off his feet and hurled him senseless against the wall.

The sharp pain in his head roused him at last. He got on his feet and tried to walk, but his knees shook so that he had to lean against the wall to avoid falling. Holding on with both hands to the wall he dragged himself to the porch.

Stumbling over heaps of brick and plaster and broken glass he staggered into the church.

The nave was dark, but early dawn lit up the choir. On the steps which had led to the high-altar, stood the priest in his chasuble celebrating morning Mass in his ruined sanctuary. Tall and erect his figure stood out against the reddening sky. "*Gloria in excelsis Deo!*" came from his lips amidst the moan from the straw-covered floor.

Gloria in excelsis Deo!

As he lifted the chalice over his head the sun rose through the broken vault of the apse to reveal to the day the dark deed of the night.

II

V

THEY came. Preceded by a couple of dusty motor-cyclists with carbines slung upon their backs hunter-fashion, they entered the village at an easy trot, tall and strong on their magnificent horses, their pennons floating in the breeze and the sunlight gleaming on their lance-tips.

The Mayor in his tricolour scarf, with the Curé at his side, stood in front of the church, but no notice seemed to be taken of them as the Uhlans rode past. Five officers, all wearing the Iron Cross, followed in the rear, and dismounting, one of them saluted stiffly and informed the Mayor in quite good French that he and his officers were to be billeted in the Presbytery and that the Mayor was to provide within two hours food for the men and forage for the horses. The Mayor answered that all eatables and forage had been requisitioned for the retreating French troops, that there was hardly any food left for the few old men, women, and children remaining in the village, and that all the hay had been used to lay under the wounded in the church.

"I give you six hours," said the officer.

"How many wounded have you got in there, and are there any officers amongst them?" asked another. "I will come and inspect them in half an hour; see that the doctor in charge is there to receive me."

They saluted and all five leisurely entered the Presbytery.

Punctually half an hour later two officers followed by an orderly came to the church.

"Are you in charge of the ambulance?" said one of them to Doctor Martin, noticing the brassard round his arm.

Before the Doctor had time to explain their terrible situation to his colleague—for he had by now realized that he had a German army-surgeon before him—the two officers had already begun their inspection.

"Show me the officers first," said the surgeon.

He pulled off their blankets, giving them each a rapid glance, and then passed along the row of soldiers, shrugging his shoulders significantly as he looked at each of them.

"Nothing for you, my dear Adalbert," said he in German, turning to the officer at his side.

"Where is the General?" he asked

abruptly. He was told there was no General amongst the wounded.

"I know your commanding General was badly wounded up in that wood. Where has he been taken to? Where is your nearest clearing hospital?"

He got no answer.

"You won't say?" insisted the German

"No."

"I fear you will go away from this place with an empty bag, my dear Adalbert," said the surgeon to his comrade. "Not one of these people is worth your trouble, not one of them would reach the frontier alive, they are all as good as gone. As for the village, there are only some old women and children left as far as I could see—unless you want to bag that hunchback who was hanging about outside the church," he added laughingly.

"How much chloroform have you got?" asked the surgeon.

"None, and no medicine, no disinfectants, and, as you can see for yourself, no dressing-material either."

"What a show! And what a stench, eh!"

"*Kolossal!*" replied Adalbert, holding tightly to the handkerchief over his nose.

"Indeed they have had a narrow escape," said the surgeon, looking towards the choir. "Had the shell struck the church only a few yards higher up the main vault would have fallen in and the whole fabric would have crumbled like a pack of cards and buried them all."

"Or one of those big wooden rafters might have caught fire and burnt them alive," suggested Adalbert. "Anyhow it is not bad as it is at ten miles range," said he, examining the broken vault through his monocle. "I am sure those old walls are over two mètres thick. They talk the whole time at the top of their voices of their famous '75's, but they are nothing but toy pistols compared to our long range guns! When I was at Potsdam . . ." He stopped short as he noticed the Doctor's eye upon him.

In a futile attempt to be polite he continued in French, turning to the Doctor:

"I was just saying to my comrade how lucky it was that the shell struck so low. Reading about it in a newspaper nobody would believe in such luck—a twelve-inch shell making a hole as big as a transport waggon, smashing the high-altar and passing clean through the nave out of the rose window over the porch, without doing any damage. It is very interesting. When I was at Potsdam . . ."

"Were you in the church when the shell struck?" asked the surgeon.

"No, I was standing outside in the middle of the chaussée, and the shell must have passed only a few mètres over my head, judging from the height it struck the wall."

"You must be born under a lucky star," complimented Adalbert, "and not even your eyes blown in. It is most interesting."

"Was anybody killed in the church?" asked the surgeon.

"No, they were all covered by falling plaster and broken glass—you can see there is not a single pane left in the windows—but none of our men were killed. They are evidently all born under the same lucky star as I."

"It is to be hoped that in the state of collapse they all are in they did not even realize their danger," said the surgeon.

"Quite so, they have nothing more to fear from life, they are safe under the protection of approaching death."

"I am very glad to hear it," said Adalbert politely. "It was one of those unfortunate accidents unavoidable in war. It must have been a stray shot whilst our battery was getting the range—I suppose you know that Fort Vendôme was bombarded just before daybreak. I hope you understand that we don't bombard churches."

"I thought you did," said the Doctor. "I was at Rheims."

The surgeon bit his lip.

"I wish you could help us to get a proper bandage and a drainage-tube for the Bavarian soldier over there," said Doctor Martin, with a superhuman effort to keep his nerves in hand.

"Why didn't you tell us you had a German here?"

"You have not given me time to tell you anything," answered Doctor Martin.

The surgeon looked unmoved at the terrible wound, and sent the orderly to fetch his instrument case and necessary dressing material, talking the while on indifferent matters with his comrade without saying a single word to the wounded man.

"*Potzdonnerwetter!* There he brings me the wrong scissors again!" shouted the surgeon, as the orderly with a stiff salute handed him the instrument case. "And what the devil am I to do with these two small rolls of bandages for a man who has his whole head almost blown off! And do you call this a drainage-tube! You d——d fool!"

"Damn you!" said Adalbert.

"It is no good wasting our time with

this confounded ass," said the surgeon, throwing the rolls of bandages at the orderly's head. "I shall have to go myself to fetch what I want or I shall never get it! I shall be back in a minute. Promise, my dear Adalbert, not to talk any nonsense," he added in a low voice in German as he walked out of the church, followed by the orderly, who looked quite placid and unconcerned.

"So you were at Rheims!" said Adalbert to the Doctor. "I must say I envy you having been there. It must have been a wonderful sight to see the huge cathedral in flames, one of those sights one can never forget."

"Never!" said the Doctor.

"Pray pardon me," said Adalbert, looking at the other through his monocle, "may I ask what that red ribbon is on your tunic? I am very much interested in decorations. Surely it is not, it cannot be, the Legion of Honour?"

"I daresay the name sounds unfamiliar to your ears, but that is what it is called."

"Really! I did not know it was so easy to get the Legion of Honour," explained Adalbert. "I thought it had been invented as a sort of equivalent, I mean substitute, for our famous Iron Cross; but with us, of course, this glorious decoration is only awarded on rare occasions for high personal valour in serving the Fatherland or for conspicuous gallantry—or both," he added, nonchalantly toying with his Iron Cross.

"Isn't that rather a good picture?" said Adalbert, staring through his monocle at an old Madonna over the side altar. "I am sure it is German; it looks like a Dürer."

"Flemish late seventeenth century, I should say," rejoined the Doctor.

"Why play with words," laughed Adalbert. "Flemish or German is all the same now. You must have very good eyes to see the date it was painted in this dim light," he added wittily.

"Yes, I have very good eyes; they are the best thing I have."

"I am sure it is a valuable picture; pity it is so large!" said Adalbert meditatively. "We are very fond of old pictures in Germany. When I was at Potsdam..." He suddenly grew very pale and put his handkerchief to his mouth. "I think I must have some fresh air," he said, apologetically. "I am not feeling very well. Let us continue our conversation outside the porch till my comrade comes back, if you do not mind. I like to talk to you."

The Doctor, who had by now classified his man as a rare and precious specimen well worthy of further study, followed the German with a twinkle in his eye. Leaning against the door Adalbert breathed the fresh air with evident delight.

"I am all right again," said he.

"So glad," said the Doctor, seating himself on the bench.

"I suppose you know who I am," said Adalbert, placing himself before the Doctor.

"I have no idea."

"I am *Graf Adalbert von und zu Schoenbein und Rumpelmayer*," announced the German. "Pray be seated," he added, with a benevolent wave of the hand "My name must be known to you."

"Would you mind saying it again and a little slower," begged the Doctor, lighting his cigarette. "Ah! yes, of course, Rumpelmayer. I have often had tea at Rumpelmayer's, both in London and in Paris, such good tea and such excellent cakes! A very good business, I am sure! Any relation of yours?"

Adalbert blushed terribly

"Our family name is closely connected with modern German history," announced Adalbert solemnly. "My father, His Excellency *Graf Hulding Adalbert von und zu Schoenbein*, was *Oberküchenmeister* to his Imperial Majesty William I."

"My name is Doctor Martin," said the Doctor, "my father . . ."

"Ah! Now I understand the feeling of sympathy I felt for you from the first, and that vague air of distinction I did not fail to notice in your appearance; of course you are of German origin, your name is pure German, and what is more you are the bearer of an old name, my dear Doctor *von* Martin. You bear the illustrious name of one of the Generals of Frederick the Great, and there is also amongst the civilians our famous Martin Luther . . ."

"Sorry to have to correct you, Graf Rumpelmayer"—Adalbert frowned a little—"but I have never heard of any German ancestry of mine, and there is no handle to my name; it is plain and simple Martin. My father . . ."

"I beg your pardon," said Adalbert; "it is of course force of habit that makes me add that so significant little prefix to the names I generally mention, all my friends being noblemen."

"My father was a blacksmith," said the Doctor.

Adalbert looked round, horrified lest the sentry should hear them.

"Never mind, Martin, who your father was," he said bravely. "I am glad to see that his son has nevertheless succeeded in making himself an honourable position in life—of course, you could never have become a German officer. To go back to what we were saying," he went on, " I am glad you mentioned Rheims. Here we have again an example of what I so appropriately called an unavoidable accident of war. I am aware that a great deal of fuss has been made about this accident by the hostile press, and I have thought a good deal about it. Luckily for us we are as innocent with regard to the bombardment of the cathedral of Rheims as we are with regard to the disturbance we unhappily caused you and your wounded last night in this little church. Our conscience is quite clear. Civilians cannot understand that the position of a battery is perforce determined by the formation of the surrounding country. The unfortunate situation of the cathedral in the very firing line of our heavy guns made it unavoidable that the old building should receive a scratch or two from the claws of the German eagle—a rather striking metaphor, if you allow me to say so. Besides, Gothic architecture has had its day, and, as the *Frankfurter Zeitung* so cleverly pointed out, the disappearance of these old monuments will only hasten the birth of new and astounding creations of

German genius and *Kultur* far outdistancing these well-meaning efforts of bygone times.

"Wait till you see our new cathedral in Berlin," Adalbert went on enthusiastically. "I shall never forget the majestic impression it made upon me when I saw it the day of its consecration. It was consecrated by the All-Highest, who made a stupendous speech . . ."

"What!" exclaimed the Doctor.

"I say it was consecrated by the All-Highest, and never has his Imperial voice sounded more omnipotent and sublime than that day."

"Well I never . . ." said the Doctor.

"I must say I like to talk to you, Martin," said Adalbert. "I was reading the other day in Bernhardi . . ."

"You read a lot?"

"I am always reading."

"Doesn't too much reading interfere somehow with your thinking?"

"Thinking!" exclaimed Adalbert. "A German officer has to act and not to think; our thinking is done by our General Staff, which has been called so aptly the brain of the army."

"And what about your feeling?"

"We don't feel anything. Clausewitz says that it deteriorates the discipline of an army, and besides it sets a bad example to the men."

"How is it that you do not belong to the General Staff?"

"That is a question I have often asked myself; but I hope I shall one day."

"So do I," said the Doctor fervently.

"What a lovely idyllic country this is," said Adalbert, looking out over the smashed house-tops of the little village at his feet towards the devastated ridge of scattered pines, down to the river with its blown-up bridge and a black cloud of smoke slowly drifting across the valley from Fort Vendôme in flames. "What a charming landscape; there is something truly German about it. I have had the good fortune to explore this part of France under the most favourable conditions," Adalbert went on. "You know there is nothing like visiting a new country on horseback. I must say I do not wonder the French like their country. So do we. Good food, excellent wine, and these stately châteaux so conveniently scattered about for our billets, so home-like and comfortable, so abundantly and thoughtfully provided with all that makes life worth living. Yes, indeed, life would be ideal here were it not for one single drawback we all feel very keenly, though I hope it is only a temporary evil. You know the people here do not like us; it is useless to try to shut one's eyes to this regrettable fact. We Germans do not dislike the French, in fact we rather like them. My detachment has just been on a punitive expedition to several small places round here, and I must say that everywhere I was painfully impressed by the sullenness of the inhabitants. Our attitude towards the French has invariably been correct. Look at me, for instance. I think I may say, without boasting, that you can look upon me as a typical German officer . . ."

"I wish to goodness you were!" exclaimed the Doctor, completely off his guard. "I wish to goodness you were, for if so the war would be over in a month."

"I thank you sincerely, Martin, for these words," said Adalbert solemnly; "it does one good to be appreciated by a loyal adversary. I was saying look at me and answer me this question: Have I not treated you, who after all I must look upon as an enemy, with unfailing tact and forbearance; have I not carefully avoided touching on any of the topics which might hurt your feelings; have I not shown you my sympathetic interest in the inconvenience we unfortunately caused you last night in this little church; have I not, in one word, behaved towards you in the manner you would expect of a Prussian officer and a German gentleman?"

"You have indeed," said the Doctor.

"I thank you, Martin; I thank you. I must say I like talking with you. Well, Martin, I have behaved in exactly the same way to everybody I came across since I entered France—to those few of my own class as well as to those of yours. And what have I gained by my urbanity? You must realize my feelings of bitterness, not to say painful resentment, when I tell you that so far you are the only person who has understood my true nature; who has listened to me without malice and has been impressed by my arguments. That is why I like to talk to you, Martin; I tell it you frankly. Why do they all dislike us? We were told that French women were rather coquettish, and not at all disinclined to a little flirtation as a pastime. I cannot say that I find them so," said Adalbert gloomily. "It is quite true they are pretty, and that there is a certain coquettish air about them, but it is not to be depended upon; they are not at all responsive. The other day I saw a rather attractive girl standing in her doorway. As I went up to give her a kiss, she snatched, with incredible rapidity, her *sabot* from her foot and hurled it at my face! Luckily for her it did not hit me—you know what the punishment is for striking a German officer! Well, nine men out of ten would have had this girl shot. I did nothing of the sort—I forgave her. All I did was to have her house put on the list of those to be burned down, and as we left I even gave her a pleasant smile as I rode past her in the street."

"Did she smile at you?" asked the Doctor.

"Not at all," said Adalbert indignantly, "she shouted a word at me I have never heard before, and which I cannot for the life of me remember."

"I wonder what it can have been," said the Doctor, looking attentively at Adalbert.

"They tell me the women of the upper classes are more amiable," Adalbert went on, "but, alas! I never see any; they are all gone away. I assure you, Martin, it makes one almost sad to wander about alone in those magnificent châteaux, to lounge in their luxurious drawing-rooms, to sleep in their soft beds, to sort all their innumerable little trinkets and souvenirs, to explore their wardrobes and drawers and handle their lovely dresses and all the dainty secrets of an elegant Frenchwoman's toilette. As one sits there alone packing some lovely *lingerie* all covered with real lace, a yearning comes over one too strong for words : one feels that one was made for love as well as for war, and that one could forgive the fair owner everything were she only to come back ! Why did she ever go away ? She does not know what she has lost by her absence !"

"She will know it when she comes back !" said the Doctor.

"Alas ! it will be too late—too late ! I shall already be gone. I shall be in Paris !"

Overflowing with tenderness Adalbert sat silent, stroking his little porcupine moustache.

"Why do you look at me like that ?" he exclaimed, waking from his dreams.

"I was thinking about that word the girl with the *sabot* said to you. It suddenly struck me . . . wasn't it *crapaud* that she said ?"

"Yes, that's the word ; how clever of you. What on earth does it mean ?"

"It means a Toad," said the Doctor, rising from his seat.

But nothing happened.

"The vulgar insults of a peasant girl cannot reach Count von Schoenbein," said Adalbert loftily. "I have forgiven her once and I forgive her again. Paris ! Paris !" he went on in rapture. "What a fascination in the very name ! Paris with its gay boulevards, its theatres, its cafés-chantants, its

Maxim, its Moulin Rouge—what a place for a garrison! Do you know Paris well?"

"Yes, fairly well. I lived there for over ten years."

"I have decided to give you my card," announced Adalbert, handing with an indescribable air of protection his card adorned by an enormous crown. "You will find it both useful and agreeable to know a German officer during your stay in Paris, and I shall be very pleased if I can do anything for you."

"I understand there has been a certain delay . . ." said the Doctor.

"Yes, our solemn entry into Paris has been somewhat delayed," admitted Adalbert, "and we know that it is the English that we have to thank for this. I told you that we liked the French, but we have always hated the English, and they have always hated us. To-day we hate them more than ever for having dared to interfere with our determination to crush France.

"Ah! perfidious Albion!" he burst forth with unexpected pathos, "how haven't you cheated us; how haven't you deceived us! You made us believe that you were fast asleep and would not hear the thunder of our guns across the Channel, and behold the mere sound of tearing a scrap of paper made you spring to your feet! You made us believe you had no men fit to fight anything but niggers, and at your bidding forth comes a whole army of polo players, clerks, and schoolboys, smilingly playing the game of life and death on the fields of Belgium and France as coolly as though playing a game of football or a cricket match on the lawns of their club at home! But, mark my words, it is their last game they are playing, these smiling youngsters in their ugly, dirty-brown khaki, who have the impudence to go on smiling even when face to face with the veterans of the Prussian Guard. Yes, it is brown now, their famous khaki, but we will see to it that it will be dyed red before long!

"Listen to the voice of the poet! Listen to our great Lissauer, whose Hymn of Hate is sung in thousands of homes in the Fatherland to-day, and is recited in the schools by our children!"

"Fine!" said the Doctor, "I like it very much. I know it well; I have often heard it sung in the London music halls.

"I have listened to your eloquent speech with great interest, Count Rumpelmayer," the Doctor went on. "I take for granted that you know Germany well, and that it is the true feeling of your country you have laid before me. But when you speak of England's feeling towards Germany, I believe you are on less safe ground. You have told me that the English hate the Germans; but I venture to tell you that I do not believe they do."

"Do you really believe they like us?" said Adalbert, his face lit up by an unexpected hope.

"No, they do not like you; but they do not hate you. They loathe you."

The surgeon was coming up the steps leading to the church, with the orderly at his heels.

"Sorry I have been so long; I was delayed by the Major," said he with an uneasy glance at the two men.

"You were quite mistaken about him," said Adalbert in a low voice in German to his comrade as they walked into the church. "He is, of course, rather common, as I saw at once by his looks, and he is rather dense, but there is no harm in him. You are quite right that he showed some inclination to be insolent when we spoke to him at first; but he climbed down at once when I got hold of him. He soon found that he was no match for me. He was immensely flattered by my talking to him, and you would have been surprised to hear how he agreed to almost everything I said. I am sure that as a matter of fact he likes us."

"My dear Adalbert," said the surgeon quite unceremoniously as they walked up to the Bavarian's bed, "I have a strong suspicion that you have again been making an ass of yourself."

The surgeon cleansed and disinfected the soldier's wound with experienced hands, and with extraordinary rapidity and skill he applied a proper dressing, whilst Adalbert climbed on to the side altar to take careful measurements of the Madonna.

"Don't move, and don't try to speak," said the surgeon as he was leaving the Bavarian, "for if you do you will bleed to death."

* *

"Poor woman!" said the surgeon, with a softness in his voice which his colleague would not have thought natural to its register. "Is it her son?"

"No, it is one of your men who died last night; but she could not have nursed him more tenderly had he been her own son."

Poor Josephine stood beside the dead boy whose face she had covered with a handkerchief—to protect him against their evil eyes, as she explained afterwards. Adalbert started as he bent over the boy's delicate features, eagerly examined the buttons of his tunic, and tearing open the coarse shirt searched for the identity disc round his neck. Holding up between his fingers a black silk ribbon with a little image of the Madonna attached to it, he exclaimed in an angry voice :

" Who has taken away his identity disc and put this ribbon on him instead ? "

Josephine, very white in the face, said it was she who had put the medallion round his neck ; but that she had taken nothing from him.

" You have," roared the officer ; " you are a thief. You have stolen his identity disc with its chain, which you thought was of silver, as it very possibly was, and very likely he may have worn something else of value as well."

" I give you my word of honour that he had nothing round his neck. I noticed it myself," said the Doctor sharply.

" Search her ! " said the officer in German, turning to the soldier behind him.

The Doctor put himself before Josephine.

" I forbid you to touch this woman," said he also in German to the advancing soldier.

" You have no orders to give here," shouted Adalbert, crimson in the face.

" And I have none to receive either," said

the Doctor, rapidly losing control over himself.

"That is what we are going to see," retorted the officer, putting a whistle to his lips.

The surgeon took him by the arm, and turning their backs on the others they spoke together in a low voice for a minute or two at the foot of the Bavarian's bed.

"I give you till to-morrow morning to find the identity disc," said the officer with a haughty look at Josephine, and putting his arm under the surgeon's they walked towards the door. He turned round once more, and looking sharply at the Doctor, said:

"Why didn't you tell us you spoke German? Have you already been in Germany?"

"Since you were kind enough to inquire a moment ago," said the Doctor, addressing himself to the German surgeon, "if anybody had been killed by your bomb, I think I had better tell you before you go that as a matter of fact one man was killed here. Unlike your comrade, I have so far failed to discover anything interesting in the wreckage of this church, but I admit that this particular case is rather interesting. I have not been able to make a regular post-mortem examination, but what I have seen confirms me in the opinion both my colleague and I had formed about him before. He cannot have died from his wound, which was, comparatively speaking, slight. Nothing but plaster and some broken glass struck him. I should be glad to have your opinion about this case," said he to the surgeon; "I wish you would have a look at him. According to my opinion the man simply died of fright."

"An Englishman!" exclaimed the surgeon, looking with surprise at the khaki-clad soldier, who lay there with his collar still turned up over his ears.

"An Englishman!" chuckled Adalbert. "No, I do not think there is any need for a consultation about the cause of this man's death. We quite believe you have had ample opportunity to study these sort of cases, and we accept your diagnosis as the right one. This is not the first Englishman who died of fright when a German shell passed over him; nor will it be the last, I am sure. You are quite right: it is indeed a very interesting case!" he added with a fresh giggle, screwing in his monocle to have a look at the hated foe, hated unto death.

"The colour and the material are well copied," said Doctor Martin, pointing to the khaki greatcoat, "but the cut is deplorable. When the war is over you will have to send your Düsseldorf tailors back to London to improve their style. You are quite welcome to secure this man for your 'bag'; he is not fit to be here, either dead or alive.

"You had better have a look at him," he added, pulling down the collar which hid the face of the spy; "maybe he is an acquaintance of yours."

"Fuchs!" murmured Adalbert, and his jaw dropped.

VI

Worn out by anxiety and fatigue, the Doctor sank down on the bench in the sacristy. The long effort to keep himself in hand had taken away his last strength, and the words of the German officer burnt like fire in his weary brain.

He wondered how the surgeon had succeeded in bringing his irascible comrade to his senses, and he tried to feel grateful to his colleague for his intervention. He almost smiled as he remembered the only word he had managed to overhear in their conversation at the foot of the Bavarian's bed. Little did this odious German know, thought he, that by calling Josephine's defender *der Engländer*, he had paid him what he considered the greatest compliment of his life.

He began to wonder how the poor Mayor and the Curé were getting on, and was just on the point of despatching Josephine for news when the nun came and reported that the Bavarian was very restless and agitated.

The Doctor found him quite altered. The expression in his eyes was altogether different and he no longer seemed to understand what the Doctor said to him. His pulse was extraordinarily rapid, and it was clear that the poor fellow was in a state of great excitement. He put his trembling hands repeatedly to his mouth as if he wanted to speak, and then pointed to the door. There was a fixed, determined intensity in his eyes, and it was evident that those eyes had something to say. The Doctor tried to concentrate all his thoughts upon reading their mute message. His own brain was too tired, and notwithstanding all his former boasting to the nun, he had to tell her that he knew no more than she did what the man meant.

"He has been like that ever since the Germans left," said Sister Philippine.

In vain the Doctor touched his eyelids, telling him he was getting so tired and his eyelids were getting so heavy, heavy, and that he was soon going to fall asleep. In vain did he order him with firm voice to close his eyes. The eyes continued to stare wide open and wild at him with the same intense fixity. In vain did he, as a last resort, remind him that the German surgeon had said he must remain very still and quiet—this last argument seemed to excite him still more, and a half-suffocated groan issued from his lacerated throat. After a while the Doctor reluctantly came to the conclusion that his presence seemed rather to agitate his poor friend than to soothe him, and he thought it wiser to leave him alone, hoping he would calm down from sheer exhaustion.

He had hardly had time to sink down again on the bench in the sacristy when Anatole rushed in wild with excitement.

"*Ah! les assassins! les assassins!*" cried he, "they have murdered Pierre. He was brought in by a patrol an hour ago; they found, sewn in the lining of his waistcoat, a letter to the Commandant of the Fort, and they said he was a spy communicating with the enemy, and they shot him in the Square in front of his mother's house. *Ah! les assassins, les assassins!* Now they are going round searching every house for food. Their Commandant says that if they don't get what they want the Mayor will have to pay a ransom of five thousand francs to-morrow morning. They have found a cask of wine in the cellar of the inn and they are all getting drunk. The Mayor asked me to tell you he dared not go away and begged you to speak to the German surgeon for him."

"Come quick!" called the nun from the door.

The Bavarian had torn away his bandage and blood was streaming from his frightful wound. The Doctor bent over him, trying in vain to compress the artery with his fingers.

"Save yourself! They are sending you prisoner to Germany to-morrow!" he hissed out in a fearful effort to clear his throat from the invading blood.

"Run for the German surgeon!" cried the doctor to Josephine. "No, don't!" he called again before she had reached the door, as a torrent of scarlet blood burst forth from the lacerated carotid artery.

"Thank you," said the Doctor, stroking him gently over the eyes. The soldier looked steadfastly at him. They understood each other again, these two. There was not even a struggle. The Bavarian closed his eyes.

"*Ah! le sang, le sang! Que Dieu punisse celui qui fait couler tant de sang!*" cried Josephine.

VII

ANATOLE had been despatched to ask the Mayor and the Curé to come as quickly as they could to talk matters over, and the Doctor had thrown himself on the mattress in the sacristy whilst waiting for them. His head was weary and he felt as though he could neither think nor act. What was he to do?

The afternoon sun shone in through the little window, and the glare on the white wall made him close his tired eyes for a moment.

"*Have—you—already—been—in—Germany?*" He started violently as he heard the voice, and opened his eyes.

The room was quite dark, but for the little oil-lamp on the table, and on the bench sat the Mayor and the Curé talking in a low voice.

"I did not hear you come," said the Doctor, springing to his feet.

"We did not want to wake you," said the Curé, "you looked so tired. You have slept like a child for a good half-hour, but I am afraid you were awakened by a nightmare."

"You have a long night's walk before you, and you were well in need of the little sleep you got," said the Mayor with his kind voice.

They said they were very sorry he was leaving, but would not hear of any other course. Everything was already arranged for his start: provisions had been put in his haversack and a boy was to take him a short cut across the hills. They were to leave as soon as it was still in the Presbytery, and he ought to reach St. ——, still believed to be held by the French, early next morning. He said he felt almost ashamed to leave his two kind friends and those poor wounded in the church.

"You know well that in a day or two there will not be one of them left there," said the Mayor, "and as to us two old men, they won't do any harm to us."

"We are in God's hands," said the Curé.

"And Josephine?" asked the Doctor.

"I have already sent word to my wife she is to sleep in our house, and stay with us as long as they are here."

Seeing his hesitation, the Mayor took out of his pocket a sealed envelope and said in a low voice:

"It is of the utmost importance that this letter from the Commandant of Fort Vendôme, which was brought to me an hour ago by an old woman, should be delivered as soon as possible to the General in command. I have nobody to send; you know what has happened to poor Pierre, and God knows what has become of the two messengers I sent before. Will you undertake to deliver the letter?"

This settled the question, and the Mayor called out for Armand. A bright-eyed, charming-looking boy appeared at the door. After having ascertained that he was quite familiar with the road, the Mayor told him to go down to old Anne to get a good supper and wait in the kitchen till he was sent for without saying a word to anybody.

"Have you got a revolver?" asked the Mayor.

"No, and I don't want one," said the Doctor. "I have seen so much blood this last week, and so many wounds, and so many deaths, that I do not think I would feel like using it even if it came to the worst. Besides, as long as I wear this"—pointing to his Red Cross brassard—"I prefer not to carry arms. If I have to choose between the two I believe I am safer with the brassard than with the revolver. As for the boy, he is too small to carry a weapon and I believe that he also is safer unarmed."

"You are right as far as the boy is concerned, but you are wrong with regard to yourself," said the Mayor. "You know as well as I do that the Germans do not respect the Red Cross either on the arm of a doctor or when flying over an ambulance. The proofs against them now are too numerous to leave any doubt as to their wanton violation of the Geneva Convention. I saw with my own eyes up in the wood a Red Cross doctor lying dead with a bayonet through his chest by the side of a soldier he was evidently just attending to—he was still holding a roll of bandages in his hand. As to the Red Cross flag, it is not many days since they shelled the ambulance in Rheims, killing seventeen wounded and three nurses. The building stands all by itself and was most easily distinguishable with its big Red Cross flag from Nogent de L'Abbesse, where their battery was placed. We all know that in modern artillery it is easy with map and compass to bombard a town quite systematically and drop the shell exactly where you want it. It was the same with our village; there were no troops here and only women and children left. They dropped the shells on us just the same for mere lust of murder and destruction. That the church escaped is no merit of theirs, for one of their shells dug a hole four mètres deep in the cemetery, and short of hands as we were we had to use it as a grave for burying our first dead.

"You heard how I scolded Anatole for abusing the Boches, but I can tell you that I could have shot one of them myself, and I am not a bloodthirsty man. Did Anatole tell you? Well, I am glad he has kept his word. I asked him not to tell it, as it would only embitter our people still more. I have read in the papers stories like this, but I have tried not to believe them. I think I had better tell it you, so that you may know what the Boches are, or at least some of them.

"We found him lying under the willows at the edge of the river; he had crawled there to get water, I suppose. He was so covered with blood and mud that it was impossible to see anything of his uniform, but he wore the Red Cross brassard on his arm. I told Anatole he might be a doctor, but I must say for the honour of our profession that as I bent over his face I said to myself that he was probably nothing of the sort, not even an orderly, but that it might be one of their usual devilish tricks to deceive us. He was big and heavy of build, with a round, close-cropped head; his face was black with smoke, powder, and dirt; he had very pale blue, almost white, angry eyes, large ears, a thin, treacherous lip and an enormous jaw—in fact, he looked the brute he was. I admit that, helpless as he lay there, he gave me a sensation of fear from the moment I saw him. He had been shot through the thigh and was bleeding a lot, and the fingers of his right hand were also shot away, luckily for us. Anatole gave me his leather belt and I wound it tightly round his leg to compress the artery whilst we were waiting for the stretcher to bring him down. He was quite conscious, but did not seem to understand our French. He muttered something in German which we could not make out, but we thought he wanted us to raise his head, so we lifted him up and leaned his back against a stone. It was evidently what he wanted, for he nodded and grinned as we did so. I noticed that he was fumbling about with his left hand as if in search of something, but I could not make out what he wanted. I was kneeling with my back towards him, and Anatole was holding his leg whilst I was putting on the bandage.

"The bullet passed just over my head. He was still pointing the revolver at us when Anatole snatched it from him. I have never been so near death, and I must say that it fairly took the wind out of me. I had hardly time to realize what had happened when another shot rang out and Anatole let fall the smoking revolver from his hand.

"He had shot the Uhlan clean through the head and the brain was all over his face. Of course, Anatole was wrong to take the law into his own hands, but surely the man deserved his fate. I suppose he knew that he was liable to be shot before any court-martial for having been caught with the Red Cross on his arm and a revolver in his pocket, and that he thought that he might just as well have a go at us before."

"Are you certain he was not delirious?" asked Dr. Martin.

"I wish I could believe that he was, but I am sure he was as clear in his head as you or I. He knew his business quite well; he wanted us to raise him up in order to get better aim at us."

"It is an ugly story," said the Doctor. "I almost wish you had not told it to me."

"The sooner you know the truth the better for you," said the Mayor. "The truth is that these people are not the same as we are; they are nothing but Huns and barbarians."

"I now know," said the Doctor, "they are not the same as we are. It has been more difficult for me than for you to learn this bitter lesson of the war; for me who have lived in their country amongst righteous men and kind-hearted women; who have drunk their wine and sung their songs. I know now that you are right, that they are not the same as we. I have done with the Germany of to-day, but not with the Germany of the past, nor, I hope, with the Germany of the future which will rise one day purified and softened from its *Götterdämmerung*.

"The country I was born in says it can maintain its peace without the loss of its honour, and be it so. But I am at war; for the individual there is no neutrality between right and wrong. Yes, I know now what they are. I have read it in letters of flame and blood in the proclamations of their Generals on the blackened walls of your peaceful villages. I have heard it cried out in prayers and curses from the lips of their victims. I have seen it in the burnt faces of a little row of angels' heads amongst the debris of the high-altar of the Cathedral of Rheims.

"You call them Huns and barbarians, I call them cool-headed, scientific criminals, guilty of horrors which have not as yet got a name in our language.

"Listen to what I saw not many days ago in a house they had just hurriedly left. Let me tell it you as I saw it, as I felt it, with its small details and its great horror. Maybe you will say I am sentimental, and maybe you are right; I suppose I was made so and it is now too late to mend.

"A broken-down motor-car of theirs still stood before the garden gate. In the hall stood two packing-cases ready for the pictures already detached from the walls. In the drawing-room the big Venetian mirror was smashed to pieces, and there was not one single chair that had not its legs broken, its brocade ripped open. In the diningroom the big table was loaded with empty champagne bottles, and the floor was strewn with broken glass and china and playingcards. In the bedroom of the mistress of the house all the wardrobes and drawers stood wide open, with all their contents flung in heaps on the floor, dresses and cloaks of muslin, silk and velvet, all torn to rags as if some sort of savage satisfaction had been derived from the harsh sound of the very tearing. Two carefully sorted piles of *lingerie* lying on the table revealed the presence of an officer—as usual the temptation to secure fine underlinen had proved irresistible to the head of the band.

"'*La chambre des enfants*,' said the old caretaker as she opened the door to the children's nursery on the top floor. The room was large and airy, the walls were white, and the setting sun shone in through the big window facing the garden. Near the door stood a rocking-horse on three legs stripped of its saddle, its mane and tail torn off, its back and flanks hacked by deep, angry cuts from some sharp instrument. In the corner of the room stood a large doll's house with its red-tiled roof smashed in, and half buried amongst the wreckage lay its tiny inhabitants amidst all sorts of broken toy furniture, diminutive chairs, sofas and cupboards, lilliputian kitchen utensils and crockery. On a low table under the window stood a musical box all knocked to pieces. In a child's swing sat a huge felt monkey with outstretched arms, stunned by a violent blow that had almost severed the head from the body. The polished floor was strewn with lacerated sheets of children's picture books and dolls and toys of every description, tin soldiers, mousquetaires, harlequins, elephants, sheep, dogs, cats and rabbits, motor-cars, aeroplanes, and captive balloons, all smashed to atoms. The gaily coloured prints on the white walls were splashed with ink. Leaning against the pillows of a little settee sat a big teddy bear with his stomach ripped open. In a dainty brass bed with blue curtains, well tucked up under her embroidered counterpane lay a smart Paris doll with her own baby doll clasped in her arms, murdered in her sleep by a well-directed blow which had battered in her face. At the foot of the bed lay a gallant little *Chasseur d'Afrique* in his wide red trousers and gold-braided tunic with both his arms torn out of their sockets.

"Over the settee where the dead teddy bear sat was a large picture of three lovely children with long curls and delicate, refined faces. Holding each other by the hand they smiled happily upon their fairy world. On the pale blue rug before the settee was the big, dirty mark of an enormous foot.

"There is a name for the treacherous invasion and the merciless pillage of a peace-loving land, and thousands of arms are raising the gallows where some day the guilty shall swing. But what is the name for the hatred that stole into this nursery, what is the expiation that awaits the unclean monster who came here to crush the laughter of these three little children under his cloven foot? How am I to classify the murderer of a doll? What unknown power of darkness led him here to this white room? Animal instinct? Certainly not, for not even the infuriated ape, sinister forerunner of primitive man, would have simulated murder in carrying out his work of wanton destruction! Human instinct? Certainly not, for not even the Hun would have destroyed the little belongings of these fugitive children, left by them in trust, in trust to what is sacred to every living man.

"'Were they drunk?' I asked the old caretaker.

"'No, I cannot say they were, at least not the men. They all drank a lot, as you may judge from the empty bottles all over the house, but I cannot say they were actually drunk. They did no harm to the house until an hour before they left, when they began to smash everything; there is hardly a single chair left unbroken.'

"'Did they steal anything?'

"'The two miniatures of the great-grand-parents of Monsieur le Comte, said to be very valuable, are missing.'

"'Where is the Count?'

"'He was dangerously wounded at Rethel and Madame la Comtesse is with him. I am her old nurse,' said she.

"'And these children?' I asked, pointing to the picture.

"'They were taken out of their beds just after midnight when the shell struck the pavilion, and dressed hurriedly by me and the English nurse. A second shell burst with a horrible glare in the stable yard just as we put them in the pony trap. They were not at all afraid; they thought it was fireworks, and they were quite happy because they thought they were going to their mother. They absolutely wanted to bring their teddy bears, but there was no time. The Countess had given orders to the nurse that the children were to be taken to the nuns at Ste Geneviève in case of any danger, but nobody dreamt then that the Germans would come here. I didn't want them to go, but the nurse said she must obey the orders of Madame la Comtesse. It is a good hour's drive from the village to the Convent. I was so anxious, and I came up here and sat in the nursery, where I felt as if they were nearer to me. I sat looking at their picture, when suddenly I thought I saw a red glare on the wall. I rushed to the window and my knees bent under me as I saw the whole village in flames, and further down the valley big fiery shells bursting over the bridge and all along the road. I stayed there till daybreak, praying God on my knees to have mercy on my little children. In the morning the son of our gardener came up from the village and said everyone had fled during the night and that hundreds had been killed on the road by the falling shells. He started at once on his bicycle for Ste Geneviève, but came back an hour later; the

Boches were holding the bridge and they had shot at him as he tried to pass. He said the whole sky was black with smoke in the direction of Ste Geneviève, and he had heard that the town had been set on fire in the night. In the afternoon the Boches came here and took possession of the house; four officers, all wearing the Iron Cross, and lots of soldiers. I asked an officer for God's sake to send somebody to inquire if the children were safe with the nuns. He did send somebody, and I could see he was ashamed when he told me next morning that Ste Geneviève was in ruins and the Convent had been destroyed by fire. I begged him to help me to send a telegram to Madame la Comtesse, but he said all the wires were cut. He said it was a folly to send the children away that night and that no harm would have come to them here.

"'Since then everybody in the Château has been out in search of them, but nobody has seen or heard anything of them, nobody knows if they are dead or alive.'

"The sun had gone down and twilight was falling over the nursery. I looked at the three children on the white wall. A weird sensation came over me that I knew these three children, that I had seen them somewhere before. Where had I seen these faces with their long curls?

"'Where are you, my poor children?' cried the old nurse, bursting into tears.

"'I shall never see my darlings any more, my angels, my angels!'

"I looked at them again as she spoke.

"Suddenly I recognized them, as I heard them called by their name. The same long curls encircled their brows, but their faces had become so white and grave in the fading light of the day. It was the little row of angels' heads from the Cathedral of Rheims that looked at me from the wall of the nursery."

VIII

The Mayor opened the drawer in the table and took out a five-chambered Browning revolver. "The country swarms with Germans, one never knows what may happen, and if your hand is as steady as your head is cool it will always help you to account for five of them if it comes to the worst."

Yielding to the insistence of the Mayor the Doctor reluctantly took the revolver and put it in his hip-pocket.

The old Doctor had just begun to explain on the map the road his colleague was to take when Anatole came to say that a soldier was at the door with a message that the Mayor was wanted by the Commandant. He took a hearty farewell of Dr. Martin, wishing him God-speed in case he should not be able to return before the start.

The Mayor having left, the Doctor took the Curé aside and told him that he would rather have Anatole than the boy as his guide.

"You do not like Anatole?" said the Curé.

"Not particularly."

"That is why you prefer to take him?"

"Yes."

"Anatole is better than you think," said the Curé, "but maybe you are right."

Anatole was delighted, and having successfully passed a rapid examination as to his knowledge of the road, he was sent down to the kitchen to get something to eat and to tell the boy he was not needed.

* *

The Doctor went into the church for his last round.

The lugubrious work, delayed by all that had happened, had been going on while he was asleep in the sacristy, and the death-harvest for the night and the day had been gathered. The *luthier*, the blind soldier, Josephine's boy, the gardener who was such a hand at flowers, the Bavarian giant who had given his life in exchange for a kind word—they were all gone, these and many others who had surrendered at last to the Invincible Foe.

"Good-bye Josephine! I have only known you for thirty-six hours, but I shall never forget you! I feel as if I wanted to give you something, Josephine, but I have got nothing to give. This is no longer of any use to me," said he, taking the brassard from his arm and handing it to her. "If ever anybody had the right to wear the Red Cross it is you, Josephine; you have in any case infinitely more right to wear it than I have. I have learnt a lot from you, Josephine, and I thank you for it!"

"How could you learn anything from me," said she, "I know so little, I can barely read and write, and you know so much, you know everything. Sister Philippine says that you even know what one thinks."

"Yes, Josephine, now and then I do know what one thinks," said the Doctor with a smile. "I am not a soldier, and in no need of an identity disc round my neck, but I am badly in need of your prayers, so why don't you give me that little image the German threw back at you, and which you are now holding between your fingers."

Josephine got quite red in the face. "How did you know, how could you know? I wanted so much to give it you, but I had not the courage to tell you. How could you know?"

"I did not know that I knew," said the Doctor simply.

* *

Sœur Marthe sat fingering her rosary at the little shrine near the door, lit up by a solitary candle.

"Who is that candle for?" asked the Doctor.

"For the greatest sinner here," said the nun. "He stands now before his Judge. His heart was full of hatred, his hands were stained with innocent blood; he needs our prayers more than anybody else if God is ever to forgive him his terrible sin."

"Yes, Sœur Marthe, he needs your prayers, but whether he needs them more than anybody else in order to be forgiven, is not known to us. God judges not in the same way as we do. He alone knows who is the greatest sinner."

"He died with the name of the Evil One upon his lips," said the nun.

"There is, I believe, a far greater sin than that: to live and sin with the name of God upon your lips. That is, I believe, the only sin which cannot be forgiven. This man dared not speak to God; he knew that he had abandoned his God, and he believed that God had abandoned him. It is this fearful thought, the thought that God has abandoned us, that we call Hell. There is no other hell.

"All the rest is God's beautiful earth, and the whole earth is all filled with His presence. Under the earth sleeps the spring amidst the seeds of the flowers to come, and deeper down, under the roots of the friendly trees, under the beds of the mighty rivers and in the hollows of the cloud-capped mountains, are nature's vast factories and storehouses, where thousands of humble lives are toiling night and day for the glory of God. Over the earth are the stars, and over the stars are still other stars, and over them is Heaven. There is no room for hell anywhere. It is in our darkest thoughts only that the devil has his realm. No, Sœur Marthe, this man won't go to hell; he has already been there, and God in His mercy has taken him out of it. He did not die; it was the devil in him we watched dying in that charnel-house."

"I do not understand," said Sœur Marthe timidly. "I have never heard anybody speak like that; I do not know if I ought to listen to you. How can you not believe in hell! Don't you know that even Our Lord descended into hell to save us from our sins. Are you . . . are you . . . a Protestant?" said she, drawing back a little.

"Dear Sister, I do not know what I am," said he, "I only know that I believe in the same God as you, and that I love your Madonna."

" Don't you pray ? "

" Alas! not so often, and not so well as you, kind Sister. I used not to believe in any other God than the God of Mercy. How could I believe in the God of Wrath—I, who have been forgiven so much and so often? Now I have lived to learn to believe that there is and must be a God of Vengeance as well. I feel as if I could not live on if I were to lose my faith in Him. Sœur Marthe, if I were to pray to-day it is to Him I would pray:

" *Stern God of Israel, whose voice amongst the thunders and lightnings upon the Mount made all the people that was in the camp tremble! Why do you tarry? There is not one of Your Commandments they have not trodden under their feet, there is not one of the gentle messages of pity Your Son gave to the world that they have not scorned. Is there not enough broken faith in their torn pledges to You and to Man, is there not enough blood on their hands? Are there not enough homeless children calling out to their fathers, are there not enough tears in the women's eyes? You used to strike hard in the days of old, avenging God of Judah, at the false prophets who said their words were Your words! Why do You remain silent now while they are calling out that they are the Chosen People of the Lord, while they are bringing down Your temples in the name of their God who is not our God, while they are wrecking Your altars with the name of another Messiah on their lips, a Messiah who cannot be Your Son who taught us to love and to forgive!*

"King of Kings! Why do not You let the thunder of Your voice be heard once more! Why do not You send down once more upon our bleeding earth that Angel of Yours 'who went out at night and smote in the camp of the Assyrians an hundred four score and five thousand, and when they arose early in the morning behold they were all dead corpses'?"

"God chooses His time," said the nun.

* *

The Doctor went back into the sacristy and sat down on the bench beside the Curé, waiting for the hour to start. All was still, and the silence was only broken by the never-ceasing moan from the church.

"I feel as if I ought not to leave these poor dying men," he said.

A roar of laughter rang through the night.

"Do you hear them?" whispered Anatole under the window. "They are having their supper in your dining-room. They are all five sitting round the table in the midst of the room; their faces are as red as turkey-cocks, and they never cease to laugh except when they empty their glasses at one gulp and put them down on the table with a bang. They all talk at the top of their voices and don't hear anything. I crept up close under the window; I was as near them as I am to you, and could have heard every word they said had I understood the Boche language.

"Do you want to see them?" said the hunchback in an uncanny whisper, as a fresh roar of laughter struck the Doctor's ears like the cut of a whip across the face.

They walked cautiously over the grass, and as they entered the garden gate he heard his own voice say:

" Five, they are five."

" Hush ! " whispered the hunchback.

They crept alongside the hedge and stood still under a tree in front of the window. The room was strongly lit up by half a dozen candles on the table, laden with bottles and the Curé's Christmas turkey in its midst. Round the table sat the five officers, all young and strong, their faces flushed with wine.

The last story must have been a good one, for a terrific outburst of laughter shook the window-panes. One of the officers stood up, bowing with grotesque gravity as though before an invisible large audience, and the voice that had called Josephine a thief began:

"When I was at Potsdam . . ."

Yells of *Hoch!* and *Prosit!* curtailed the peroration, and the speaker sat down amidst a fearful banging of instantaneously emptied glasses.

Then another rose with a stiff bow and with equal gravity the voice, that maybe an hour before had ordered Pierre to be shot, began:

"*Gott strafe England!*"

The Doctor looked on fascinated. Compelled by an invisible force he drew nearer and nearer till at last he stood motionless, leaning against the window-sill. His eyes stared wide open and still on the five men. He heard their words as clearly as if he had been in the room, but he no longer understood their meaning.

One—two—three—four—five—yes, they were five, just five. The candles on the table were also five—why five? The buttons on the surgeon's tunic were also five. Why just five? The swords standing there in the corner, were they four or five? Why didn't they wear their swords? Why didn't they have their revolvers in their leather belts? Why didn't somebody come and tell them quick to get hold of their revolvers? Why didn't Anatole go and tell them?

"Why do you want them to fetch their revolvers?" he heard a voice, his own voice, say. "Do you think that Pierre had a revolver to defend himself when they came to kill him?"

Something sinister and evil flashed suddenly through his unconscious brain like the big shell that had passed him in the darkness hurling death through the night. He felt the same grip of unspeakable fear round his throat, and with a violent effort he drew his clenched hand from his pocket and sprang out of the garden. As he opened the gate the window was flung open and a rich and melodious voice sang in the night Schubert's immortal serenade:

> *Leise flehen meine Lieder*
> *Durch die Nacht zu dir,*
> *In den stillen Hain hernieder,*
> *Liebchen komm zu mir.*
> *Flüsternd schlanke Wipfel rauschen*
> *In des Mondes Licht, in des Mondes Licht.*

"Where have you been?" asked Josephine in the porch, anxiously scrutinizing his face. "You are so pale."

"Where — have — I — been?" said he,

slowly repeating her words as if trying to understand their meaning.

"Josephine, I have been in hell!" said he, staggering into the church.

* *

The Curé and the Doctor sat silent on the bench in the sacristy. The priest's head was bent, and his eyes were fixed on the floor where the nuns had reverently deposited the broken limbs of the crucifix.

"They have killed your Christ," said the Doctor bitterly. "Is God also dead?"

"How dare you speak thus," said the Curé, lifting his head with shining eyes. "Yes, Christ was put to death by the evil in man, and His side was pierced by the soldier's lance; but He has risen again to save the world. God lives forever: His life has no beginning and no ending. He is Eternity. He is Life Itself. You and I will die, maybe to-day, maybe to-morrow; but Life cannot die—God cannot die. He is watching over us as long as we live, and when we are dead He is watching over us still. He is with us now; it was He who stayed your hand..."

The other shuddered from head to foot.

"How did you know?" said he, wiping

the cold perspiration from his forehead. " I did not know you were there."

" I stood by your side at the window."

" Did you . . . ? "

The two men looked at each other. The priest's face was livid. He bent his head again towards the crucifix on the floor.

" Did you . . . ? "

" Yes—may God forgive me," said the priest.

* *

" The wind is rising," said the Curé, looking out through the open window ; " the stars are coming out ; the night will be cold and clear."

" I am glad the stars are coming out, I shall feel less lonely on the road," said the Doctor.

" Listen to the wind sweeping down from the hills and rushing through the poplars along the chaussée ! It sounds like the voice of a mighty river rolling on towards us."

" Are you sure it is the wind ? It sounds like . . ."

They heard rapid footsteps on the grass, and Anne's voice called out under the window :

" They are off ! The Boches are off ! "

They rushed out and reached the porch in

time to see the five officers spring to their saddles and gallop down the village street.

They stood still and listened.

The storm came thundering along, nearer and nearer, gradually growing into a rhythmic roar like angry waves breaking against the rocks. Suddenly the night resounded with the furious beating of thousands of horses' hoofs against the hard pavement of the chaussée!

"Cavalry! Cavalry!" cried the Curé, lifting his hands to heaven.

The Mayor in his tricolour scarf, with the Curé at his side, stood in front of the church.

"*Vive la France!*" he called out, as line after line of stalwart cuirassiers galloped past *ventre à terre*, their steel breastplates glistening in the dark and their black *crinières* floating in the wind.

"*Vive la France!*" the men joyously called back, leaning forward on their foaming horses.

"Yes! *Vive la France!*"

* *

The Doctor went back into the church.

"No, nobody has stirred," said the nun, "they are all just the same; they don't seem to mind anything. The trooper over there, whom you said would not live through the day, just opened his eyes as the bugle sounded, but he closed them again. The lance-corporal is spitting blood, a whole pailful, and it is all over his bed. Josephine is sitting with him."

"*Ah! le sang, le sang! Que Dieu punisse celui qui fait couler tant de sang!*"

Also from Benediction Books ...

Wandering Between Two Worlds: Essays on Faith and Art
Anita Mathias
Benediction Books, 2007
152 pages
ISBN: 0955373700

Available from www.amazon.com, www.amazon.co.uk
www.wanderingbetweentwoworlds.com

In these wide-ranging lyrical essays, Anita Mathias writes, in lush, lovely prose, of her naughty Catholic childhood in Jamshedpur, India; her large, eccentric family in Mangalore, a sea-coast town converted by the Portuguese in the sixteenth century; her rebellion and atheism as a teenager in her Himalayan boarding school, run by German missionary nuns, St. Mary's Convent, Nainital; and her abrupt religious conversion after which she entered Mother Teresa's convent in Calcutta as a novice. Later rich, elegant essays explore the dualities of her life as a writer, mother, and Christian in the United States-- Domesticity and Art, Writing and Prayer, and the experience of being "an alien and stranger" as an immigrant in America, sensing the need for roots.

About the Author

Anita Mathias was born in India, has a B.A. and M.A. in English from Somerville College, Oxford University and an M.A. in Creative Writing from the Ohio State University. Her essays have been published in The Washington Post, The London Magazine, The Virginia Quarterly Review, Commonweal, Notre Dame Magazine, America, The Christian Century, Religion Online, The Southwest Review, Contemporary Literary Criticism, New Letters, The Journal, and two of HarperSanFrancisco's The Best Spiritual Writing anthologies. Her non-fiction has won fellowships from The National Endowment for the Arts; The Minnesota State Arts Board; The Jerome Foundation, The Vermont Studio Center; The Virginia Centre for the Creative Arts, and the First Prize for the Best General Interest Article from the Catholic Press Association of the United States and Canada. Anita has taught Creative Writing at the College of William and Mary, and now lives and writes in Oxford, England.

"Yesterday's Treasures for Today's Readers"

Titles by Benediction Classics available from Amazon.co.uk

Religio Medici, Hydriotaphia, Letter to a Friend, Thomas Browne

Pseudodoxia Epidemica: Or, Enquiries into Commonly Presumed Truths, Thomas Browne

Urne Buriall and The Garden of Cyrus, Thomas Browne

The Maid's Tragedy, Beaumont and Fletcher

The Custom of the Country, Beaumont and Fletcher

Philaster Or Love Lies a Bleeding, Beaumont and Fletcher

A Treatise of Fishing with an Angle, Dame Juliana Berners.

Pamphilia to Amphilanthus, Lady Mary Wroth

The Compleat Angler, Izaak Walton

The Magnetic Lady, Ben Jonson

Every Man Out of His Humour, Ben Jonson

The Masque of Blacknesse. The Masque of Beauty,. Ben Jonson

The Life of St. Thomas More, William Roper

Pendennis, William Makepeace Thackeray

Salmacis and Hermaphroditus attributed to Francis Beaumont

Friar Bacon and Friar Bungay Robert Greene

Holy Wisdom, Augustine Baker

The Jew of Malta and the Massacre at Paris, Christopher Marlowe

Tamburlaine the Great, Parts 1 & 2 AND Massacre at Paris, Christopher Marlowe

All Ovids Elegies, Lucans First Booke, Dido Queene of Carthage, Hero and Leander, Christopher Marlowe

The Titan, Theodore Dreiser

Scapegoats of the Empire: The true story of the Bushveldt Carbineers, George Witton

All Hallows' Eve, Charles Williams

The Place of The Lion, Charles Williams

The Greater Trumps, Charles Williams

My Apprenticeship: Volumes I and II, Beatrice Webb

Last and First Men / Star Maker, Olaf Stapledon

Last and First Men, Olaf Stapledon

Darkness and the Light, Olaf Stapledon

The Worst Journey in the World, Apsley Cherry-Garrard

The Schoole of Abuse, Containing a Pleasaunt Invective Against Poets, Pipers, Plaiers, Iesters and Such Like Catepillers of the Commonwelth, Stephen Gosson

Russia in the Shadows, H. G. Wells

Wild Swans at Coole, W. B. Yeats

A hundreth good pointes of husbandrie, Thomas Tusser

The Collected Works of Nathanael West: "The Day of the Locust", "The Dream Life of Balso Snell", "Miss Lonelyhearts", "A Cool Million", Nathanael West

Miss Lonelyhearts & The Day of the Locust, Nathaniel West

The Worst Journey in the World, Apsley Cherry-Garrard

Scott's Last Expedition, V1, R. F. Scott

The Dream of Gerontius, John Henry Newman

The Brother of Daphne, Dornford Yates

The Poetry of Architecture: Or the Architecture of the Nations of Europe Considered in Its Association with Natural Scenery and National Character, John Ruskin

The Downfall of Robert Earl of Huntington, Anthony Munday

Clayhanger, Arnold Bennett

The Regent, A Five Towns Story Of Adventure In London , Arnold Bennett

The Card, A Story Of Adventure In The Five Towns , Arnold Bennett

South: The Story of Shackleton's Last Expedition 1914-1917, Sir Ernest Shackketon

Greene's Groatsworth of Wit: Bought With a Million of Repentance, Robert Greene

Beau Sabreur, Percival Christopher Wren

The Hekatompathia, or Passionate Centurie of Love, Thomas Watson

The Art of Rhetoric, Thomas Wilson

Stepping Heavenward, Elizabeth Prentiss

Barker's Delight, or The Art of Angling, Thomas Barker
The Napoleon of Notting Hill, G.K. Chesterton

The Douay-Rheims Bible (The Challoner Revision)

Endimion - The Man in the Moone, John Lyly

Gallathea and Midas, John Lyly,

Mother Bombie, John Lyly

Manners, Custom and Dress During the Middle Ages and During the Renaissance Period, Paul Lacroix

Obedience of a Christian Man, William Tyndale

St. Patrick for Ireland, James Shirley

The Wrongs of Woman; Or Maria/Memoirs of the Author of a Vindication of the Rights of Woman, Mary Wollstonecraft and William Godwin

De Adhaerendo Deo. Of Cleaving to God, Albertus Magnus

Obedience of a Christian Man, William Tyndale

A Trick to Catch the Old One, Thomas Middleton

The Phoenix, Thomas Middleton

A Yorkshire Tragedy, Thomas Middleton (attrib.)

The Princely Pleasures at Kenelworth Castle, George Gascoigne

The Fair Maid of the West. Part I and Part II. Thomas Heywood

Proserpina, Volume I and Volume II. Studies of Wayside Flowers, John Ruskin

The Endeavour Journal of Sir Joseph Banks. Sir Joseph Banks

Christ Legends: And Other Stories, Selma Lagerlof; (trans. Velma Swanston Howard)

Chamber Music, James Joyce

Blurt, Master Constable, Thomas Middleton, Thomas Dekker

Since Yesterday, Frederick Lewis Allen

The Scholemaster: Or, Plaine and Perfite Way of Teachyng Children the Latin Tong, Roger Ascham

The Wonderful Year, 1603, Thomas Dekker

Waverley, Sir Walter Scott

Guy Mannering, Sir Walter Scott

Old Mortality, Sir Walter Scott

The Knight of Malta, John Fletcher

The Double Marriage, John Fletcher and Philip Massinger

Space Prison, Tom Godwin

The Home of the Blizzard Being the Story of the Australasian Antarctic Expedition, 1911-1914, Douglas Mawson

Wild-goose Chase , John Fletcher

If You Know Not Me, You Know Nobody. Part I and Part II, Thomas Heywood

The Ragged Trousered Philanthropists, Robert Tressell

The Island of Sheep, John Buchan

Eyes of the Woods, Joseph Altsheler

The Club of Queer Trades, G. K. Chesterton

The Financier, Theodore Dreiser

Something of Myself, Rudyard Kipling

Law of Freedom in a Platform, or True Magistracy Restored, Gerrard Winstanley

Damon and Pithias, Richard Edwards

Dido Queen of Carthage: And, The Massacre at Paris, Christopher Marlowe

Cocoa and Chocolate: Their History from Plantation to Consumer, Arthur Knapp

Lady of Pleasure, James Shirley

The South Pole: An account of the Norwegian Antarctic expedition in the "Fram," 1910-12. Volume 1 and Volume 2, Roald Amundsen

A Yorkshire Tragedy, Thomas Middleton (attrib.)

The Tragedy of Soliman and Perseda, Thomas Kyd

The Rape of Lucrece. Thomas Heywood

Myths and Legends of Ancient Greece and Rome, E. M. Berens

In the Forbidden Land, Henry Savage Arnold Landor

Illustrated History of Furniture: From the Earliest to the Present Time, Frederick Litchfield

A Narrative of Some of the Lord's Dealings with George Müller Written by Himself (Parts I-IV, 1805-1856), George Müller

The Towneley Cycle Of The Mystery Plays (Or The Wakefield Cycle): Thirty-Two Pageants, Anonymous

The Insatiate Countesse, John Marston.

Spontaneous Activity in Education, Maria Montessori.

On the Art of Writing, Sir Arthur Quillaer-Couch

The Well of the Saints, J. M. Synge

The Little World of Don Camillo, Giovanni Guareschi

and many others…